START LIVING

STOP DYING

Ten Steps to Natural Health

by

Mark E. Laursen, M.D., A.B.H.M.

www.NaturalBodyHealth.com

888-NATRLMD (888-628-7563)

866-XTRALIFE (866-987-2543)

Copyright Notice 2007

Published in Georgia in the United States of America

Contact: Tybee Island, Georgia, 31328

P. O. Box 926

ISBN # 978-0-9799284-0-6

0-9799284-0-0

This book is dedicated to my sons James Dennis, Jacob Aaron, Justin Ryan, David Nguyen and Matthew Christopher. Also to my daughters Kathleen Marie and Kristina Leigh.

A special thanks to Kathleen Tuten.

I would like to thank my wife Kathy for her excellent reviews and support in the development of this book.

I would like to acknowledge the final edit of this book by Ms. Judith Kern.

I would also like to thank Tom Goelitz for his initial editorial work.

Cover by Ms. Suzanne Bray.
Illustrated by Stacy and David Nguyen.

It is difficult to separate the different sources of this book: life experience, education and intuition, but certainly this book would not be possible were it not for the grace and intelligence of my friend John Williams.

It is my experience when you follow the 10 Steps to Natural Health, you can take 20 years off your biological age. You can be 70 and feel like 50; 60 and look like 40; 50 and be like 30. Using nature and what is natural as a guide, you can improve your quality of life.

Start Living

CONTENTS

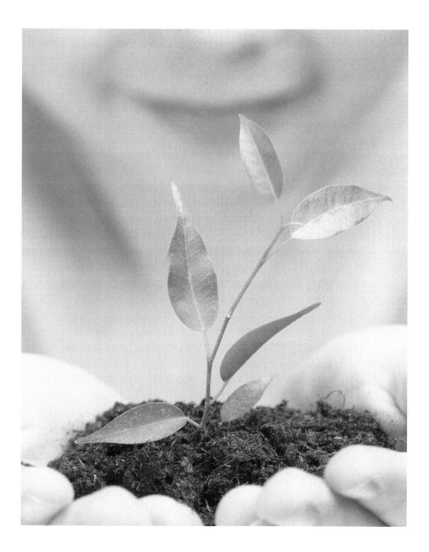

Achieving Good Health the Way Nature Intended

I am a traditionally trained medical doctor with an MD degree from the University of Iowa medical school, and yet I have chosen to complete additional training in order to become board certified in holistic medicine (2002) and completing two years of further naturopathic training in 2003. In 2004, I was the only MD, ABHM, NMD in the United States.

My traditional medical education has given me knowledge of the most up-to-date scientific methods and modalities while my holistic and naturopathic training have taught me to recognize the integrity of the whole person, the inherent healing capacity of the individual, and the ultimate responsibility of the patient for his or her own well being.

I treat patients on a mental and emotional as well as a physical level, and I am acutely aware of the degree to which these three aspects of what it means to be a human being interact. They impact one another on an everyday basis and contribute to the state of our overall health—or lack thereof.

Medical breakthroughs have virtually eliminated many of the diseases that plagued our ancestors, and yet, sadly, the more scientifically and technologically advanced our society has become, the farther we have strayed from our ancestors' fundamental natural wisdom, and the less healthy we are today. In fact, for the first time in modern history, the National Institute of Health has predicted that life expectancy for people living in industrialized societies will actually be declining, and my personal experience has led me to believe this is true.

Luckily, however, it's a lot easier to get back to living the way nature intended than it was to develop all the chemicals, toxins, artificial processed foods, and synthetic medications that were intended to improve our lives but have, in fact, been leading us astray. Nutritional supplements, herbal remedies, prescription medications, and modern technology can certainly enhance our health and well-being, but only if we use them in balance with a natural way of living and eating, thinking and feeling that is the basis of true health.

By following the ten simple steps outlined in this book you will start to heal on all levels. You will begin to stop eating artificial, processed foods and start eating naturally and according to season; you will stop eating foods that are incompatible with your unique body type and may, therefore, be making you sick; you will stop dieting because you will naturally achieve your ideal, healthy weight; you will stop buying synthetic junk supplements and start buying quality ones; stop using herbal remedies incorrectly; stop having to take so many prescription medications. You will start walking and getting other exercise. You will start to consider your lifestyle and how it is impacting your health. Most importantly, you will start to understand how your thoughts and emotions impact your physical well being. And, finally, you will start to think about fasting as the natural way to cleanse and jump-start your system so that you can gain control of your life, health, and weight.

Once you understand how great an impact these ten steps can have on every aspect of your life, and once you begin to implement them for yourself, you will be empowered to manage your own health. You will be in control of your destiny. You will start living and stop dying.

The Keys to Self-Manage & Balance your Life

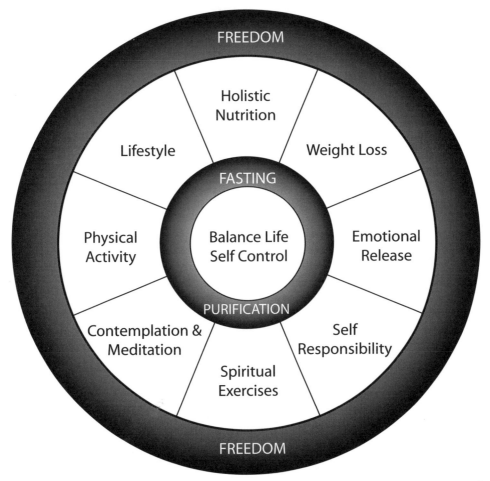

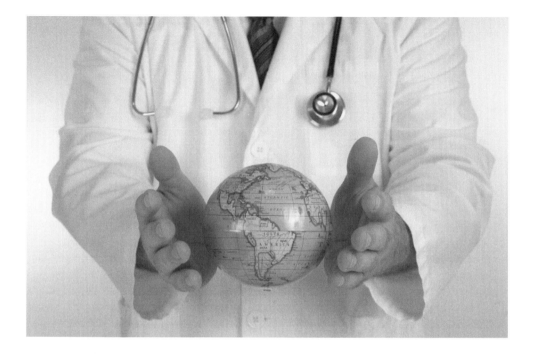

**The percentage of Americans using prescribed mind
and mood controlling drugs is historical in
perspective and evolutionary in scale.**

4

Chapter One

Health Crisis in America

Americans are spending more and more money on health care every year, and yet, according to the World Health Organization, the United States has now sunk to 37th in the world in terms of our quality of health. An astonishing percentage of children and adults are taking mind or mood altering prescription medications and the number of people diagnosed with depression, chronic anxiety, chronic pain, ADD, ADHD, sleep disorders, and stress-related stomach ailments has grown to staggering proportions. Additionally, more than one in four people is on some kind of low carbohydrate diet and yet obesity is now the second leading cause of death in the country and may soon climb to number one.

In light of this pervasive health crisis you need to consider: Are you really happy? Are you living your life with a purpose, and are you healthy enough to enjoy it? If your answer to any of these questions is no, I'm here to tell you that it doesn't have to be that way. You can reevaluate your life, take responsibility for it, and live it to the fullest. You can have more happiness on a daily basis and return your body to its ideal weight. By making just a few simple nutritional and lifestyle changes you can do away with antidepressants and other mood-altering substances and begin to live naturally.

The Trouble with Science and Technology

Modern technology has made all foods abundantly available to us, but that also means we can eat all foods all year round, even when they aren't in season. It also gives us the freedom to make too many unhealthy choices and to eat as much as we want, which, more often than not, is too much. Technology has also brought with it air pollution, impure water, and chemicals in the food supply that are acting like poisons in our bodies. Heavy metal toxicity, chronic fatigue and environmental chemical allergies are all modern illnesses.

Ironically, among the most prevalent sources of toxins in the body are the medicines we take in such excessive quantities to treat what are uniquely modern complaints. The statistics are frightening: At least 10 percent of the American population meets the criteria for major depression; 2 percent of the population is taking medication to control panic disorder and chronic anxiety; 10 percent of our children take medications for ADD, ADHD, or autism; 70 percent of us complain of sleep disorders and 15 to 20 percent rely on medication to get us to sleep. What this means is that a substantial portion of the population functions every day of their lives under the influence of drugs—and that's without considering alcohol and tobacco or illegal drugs like heroin, cocaine, and crystal meth-amphetamine.

And, if those numbers aren't scary enough, consider the following: 25 to 30 percent of Americans have stress-related ailments like ulcers,

GERD (gastroesophageal reflux disease), or upset stomach, and 56 percent of them take medication to control their symptoms. Millions more take medication for arthritis, joint pain, and muscle aches.

In fact, we have strayed so far from the natural path to healthy living that most of us are resigned to the ongoing symptoms of disease. We are ill at ease rather than happy most of the time, but rather than being alarmed by our physical aches and pains or our mental and emotional distress, we consider them normal. And why shouldn't we? The chances are that most of the people we know are suffering similar problems.

Certainly it's easier and quicker to pop a pill and receive immediate relief from our symptoms than it is to make the permanent changes that would lead to optimum health and well being over time. But as we continue down the road we've been traveling, paying less and less attention to good nutrition and relying more and more heavily on medications, our natural defenses will become even weaker, the medications we're taking will become less effective, and the bacteria and viruses that cause so many of our physical problems will become resistant to the drugs. This then becomes a vicious cycle of creating newer, stronger drugs, taking them more frequently, and increasing the toxins that are undermining our already weakened systems. The pharmaceutical industry is thriving, and the way we're headed, it will remain a growth industry for years to come.

By resigning ourselves to treating our symptoms and feelings without trying to uncover the real source of our dis-ease, we are really sabotaging ourselves. We are going for the easy quick fix to take the physical or emotional pain away. In the long run, however, the drugs we take will enslave us, and new drugs, along with new chemical alterations in our foods, will only lead us to more ill health.

The problem is that most people are so used to feeling somewhat uncomfortable so much of the time that they don't even consider they might have a health problem until it becomes an emergency. Many of our most life-threatening diseases, including heart disease, cancer, Parkinson's disease, diabetes, and Alzheimer's disease—not to mention obesity— develop over a period of many years, but their initial symptoms may be very subtle, and the farther we get from listening to our bodies the less likely we are to recognize them.

As a way to begin getting back in touch with yourself, consider the following questions.

Were you hungry before you ate your last meal?
If not, you ate for the wrong reason. Perhaps you ate out of habit, the need for pleasure, to relieve stress, or simply out of boredom. If so, you're not alone. Eating is one of the most popular forms of entertainment in our society. And even when we're engaged in other forms of entertainment, we're often also eating without even thinking about it. But eating for any

reason other than hunger is a diversion from the natural path and often leads to ill health or becoming overweight.

Do you read food labels or pay attention to the source of your food?
If not, you are undoubtedly consuming toxins, poisons, and incompatible foods that will damage your mind as well as your body. Additives are so pervasive in our food supply that even those foods that are apparently wholesome and healthy often contain toxic substances. In truth, even three of the most recommended "health foods"—namely unfermented soy, canola oil, and seafood—can act as poisons in the body. You'll be hearing more about these in the following chapters, but for now suffice it to say that if you don't know what to avoid and you're not reading labels, what you eat may slowly be eating away at your health.

Do you go to bed feeling exhausted?
Tiredness isn't just about physiology; it's about attitude, too. If your mind is focused on being tired when you go to bed, you will be entering the sleep cycle with an overburdened and fatigued mental system that struggles to find rest and peace. If you're not being restored by getting a good night's rest, you will then wake up tired, and your body will be dealing with unresolved emotional toxins that can affect your entire day. If you don't awake rested, you are becoming ill.

Think about those nights when you've gone to bed feeling content and happy. You undoubtedly awoke earlier the next morning because you felt rested with less sleep. There are ways to "dump" leftover negative thoughts and emotions at bedtime and improve the quality of your sleep. We'll be talking more about those in Chapter Six, Healing Emotional Exercises.

Do you fall asleep easily?

If, like an estimated one third of the population, you don't sleep well, there is something wrong with the types of foods you're eating and the way your mind is functioning. Eliminating foods that are incompatible with your genetics and engaging in some simple self-inquiry to understand and change the way your mind is working can help you sleep better.

What is the first thought that comes into your mind upon awakening? If you wake up thinking about a problem, that's probably something you need to work on. If it's a joyful thought, it's probably telling you where you should be directing your energy that day. Man's natural state is to be happy and enthusiastic, so if you rarely wake up feeling enthusiastic about the day ahead, your body and mind are probably out of balance.

Perhaps you have too much on your plate; perhaps you should consider whether your chosen occupation is actually bringing you fulfillment; or perhaps poor nutrition has taken its toll on your spirit.

Do you tend to feel more unhappy than happy?

Are you positive or pessimistic? Are your thoughts of other people kind or critical? It's natural to feel down once in a while, and all of us may mentally insult even the people we love at one time or another. But the way we think of others tends to reflect the way we think about ourselves. Negative thinking has a direct, toxic effect on our body and can be a primary cause of illness.

Do you use antidepressants, narcotics, or anti-anxiety medications?
If so, you are masking your symptoms with prescription medications and inhibiting the clarity you need to determine the original cause of your depression or anxiety. By doing that, you are making it more difficult to create the mental healing that will also lead to improved physical health.

Do you have a bowel movement ten to thirty minutes after finishing a meal?
If not, your elimination and detoxification systems are overburdened. Your body is quite likely reacting to incompatible or toxic foods that are causing it to back up and become constipated. The longer your body retains the waste it needs to eliminate the more you are also overloading your other detoxification systems—the lungs, kidneys, liver, and skin.

Where Real Happiness Lies

Modern society has created a matrix of unrealistic and unfulfilling beliefs—our possessions validate our worth; it's shameful to grow old; relationships are disposable; we are required to be beautiful, and so on—that make it hard to get in touch with our true nature and notice the core thoughts that motivate our actions. As a result, many of us, to a greater or lesser degree, sabotage the very things that could really be making us happy.

Perhaps the most fundamental source of overall happiness is the food we eat. What we eat has a direct effect on how we think, our emotional well being, and how our bodies feel—in fact, every aspect of our "self," which is comprised of body, mind, and spirit. And yet, our basic food supply is now so unnatural and contaminated that a recent study done by Mount Sinai Hospital in New York City found an average of ninety-one foreign chemicals in the systems of the people tested. So-called scientific and technological "advances" as well as the economic impetus toward high production and increased shelf-life have destroyed our ecology and poisoned our minds and our bodies. So, although we certainly have all the resources we need to lead happy, healthy lives, we face an onslaught of physical, mental, and emotional crises from making poor choices.

When it comes to eating, less can be more. In fact, the one factor most consistently linked to living longer is eating less. Unfortunately, however, to most people that means "going on a diet," which they associate with being deprived. People equate dieting with suffering and fail to uncover the negative thoughts and feelings that led them to overeat and become overweight in the first place. They don't understand that they were "suffering" before they began dieting.

Instead of going on—and then off—a restrictive diet that probably isn't healthy to begin with, we need techniques that will help us to balance thoughts and emotions and a natural, holistic-minded nutritional plan to cleanse and maintain our bodies. When we choose to eat chemical-laden foods, we can expect physical discomfort to follow. While this may be uncomfortable for us, it's our body's way of trying to cleanse itself of the toxins we've introduced with our food. We might experience vomiting or diarrhea or run a fever to purge our system, or we might have a complete loss of appetite so that our body can stop more bad stuff from coming in while it deals with the bad stuff that's already there.

In fact, fasting, as you'll be learning in the chapters that follow, is one of the most beneficial and natural ways there is to cleanse your body and rebalance your thoughts and emotions. Not only does fasting burn fat in the same way as popular low carb diets—but more quickly and efficiently and without their potentially dangerous side effect—but it also heightens awareness and gives us new insight into ourselves.

How to Take Control of Your Health

The original Latin meaning of the word "physician" is teacher, but these days it's highly unlikely that a physician will teach anything to his patients. More likely he or she will spend about fifteen minutes with a patient, prescribe a medication, and then move on to the next patient. And even if they did spend more time with their patients, most doctors don't really understand the importance of nutrition, nor do they appreciate the effects of toxicity upon the body, mind, and emotions, because these are not things they're taught in medical school. But what physicians don't teach you, you can learn for yourself.

As you begin to take control of your own health and well being, the one golden rule you can count on is that what is natural is generally best. The foods created by Mother Nature are usually better than the ones man has synthesized from chemicals. If you stop to think about it, nature has the evolutionary edge. In terms of the history of humanity, we've been manufacturing foods for a very short time. Our bodies have evolved with the foods nature has supplied, which means that they are likely to be more compatible with health. The apple that fell on Newton's head would tend to be more compatible with our bodies than a Fig Newton. The cherries on George Washington's ill-fated tree are probably better for us than a cherry Pop Tart. And the three bears' porridge is undoubtedly a better breakfast than a Slim Fast bar or shake.

Beyond that, however, the foods that are native to the geographical area of your ancestors are those most likely to be compatible with your genetic predisposition. They are, in other words, more *natural* for you than foods that grew in other parts of the world and were, therefore, not available to your ancestors.

But not all natural substances are good for us. Caffeine,

14

monosodium glutamate (MSG), and very long chain oils such as cottonseed and canola oils, are not healthy for anyone. And sugar, which would not be so damaging if we ate it in small amounts, becomes unhealthy in the quantities most Americans consume it. You'll be learning more about all these and other good and bad foods in the pages that follow.

Fortunately, however, all of us are born with a healing intelligence that works outside the realm of intellect. You may call it intuition or common sense. Some people call it the spiritual brain. Whatever name you give it, however, it's the healing system within us that lets us know we need more sleep or that drives us to crave certain foods when our bodies need the particular nutrients they contain.

Unfortunately modern science, and particularly modern medicine, has ignored this inner healing knowledge. For science, if something can't be measured, it doesn't exist, and since the mind can't be quantified, science tends to ignore its power. Furthermore, our reliance upon science to cure our mental and physical woes has led us to ignore the importance of the human spirit. But sadly, ignoring any reality for long enough inevitably leads to complications. And this is particularly true when what we're ignoring is the power of the mind to affect the body.

If we're dealing with a bacterial infection or the pain of a broken bone, medications will generally be effective, but if what we're medicating is mental or emotional pain, the effect is not the same at all. Beyond that, however, it is also necessary to understand what mental or emotional condition has led to the physical illness. Sometimes life can be so stressful that people subconsciously manifest illness from the inside out just to get a reprieve. With antidepressants they can remain happily unhealthy. But antidepressants are not a cure, and if they stop taking their medication, the symptoms of depression will return. If depression is within you, only you can cure it by looking within for its cause so that you can let it go. It was you who manifested the problem in all its complexity, and it is you who can manifest the solution.

Natural Health is the Way to Permanent Weight Loss

Given the obesity epidemic in the United States today, it would be impossible to talk about health without discussing the issue of weight loss. Achieving and maintaining an ideal body weight is much more than a matter of looking good or improving self-esteem. In terms of health, being overweight is associated with many debilitating and even life-threatening illnesses including high blood pressure, diabetes, arthritis, and heart disease, and may be the risk factor most closely associated with diminished longevity and quality of life.

In fact, even the "ideal" weight currently being recommended by health experts is about 5 percent more than what would be truly ideal. In my opinion, the best body weight for most people, with some genetic variations, is thin—approximately 9 to 12 percent body fat for adult men and 12 to 15 percent for most adult women. Anything above these figures puts you at increased risk for one or more of the various conditions cited above.

Despite the constant barrage of media attention to weight and the millions of dollars being made every year by the weight loss industry, no diet has ever been proved to work for most people for any length of time. If there were a quick-fix approach to weight loss that worked, it would have been discovered by now. But because there are so many factors— including stress, lifestyle, and unbalanced thoughts and emotions— involved in becoming overweight, "fixing" the problem requires a multifaceted approach as well. The only true path to permanent weight loss is the type of holistic healing approach that I take with my patients and that you will be learning by following the ten steps I lay out in the following chapters.

Although obesity is now considered a disease in and of itself, it is actually a result of other, probably several, originating diseases—diseases of the mind (how we think), diseases of the emotions (how we manifest and repeat harmful emotions), diseases of nutrition (eating wrong or incompatible foods); and diseases of lifestyle (wrong habits and activities that lead to overeating).

Food and lifestyle are the major physical causes contributing to overweight and obesity, but mental and emotional causes are also supremely important because, as I've said, we are comprised of body, mind, and spirit, all of which must be in balance in order to have good health. The correlation between the number of people who are overweight and those who are also taking mood- or mind-altering medications should be convincing evidence of the fact that obesity can and does develop as the result of a stressful lifestyle. How much you weigh can often be directly related to how you work, how you spend your free time, how you create or express yourself *or not*, and whether *or not* you live a passionate, balanced life.

Addictions and cravings are the body-based emotional and chemical drives that result from feeling that we "need" something. What we really need, however, is to generate more positive emotions, thoughts, and feelings. Once you discover the past influences that are the source of your negative thoughts and emotions you will be able to change and correct them. I'll be providing techniques in the Healing Emotional Exercises chapter that will help you to do that and to recapture your natural feelings of joy, openness, and enthusiasm.

Because the ten steps outlined in the following chapters address your overall well being on a holistic—physical, mental, and emotional—level, they will lead you naturally to healing on every level, including a healthy body weight.

Think Yourself Healthy

Your lifestyle is the result of your beliefs and emotional drives, and if you change them you will change yourself. Most people have thought themselves ill sometime in their past. Applying the knowledge you'll find in this book will help you to change that. Managing your own health and taking responsibility for your own life will give you the true reward of freedom.

No on-again-off-again diet will fix you. Medications for reflux, sleeplessness, ulcers, depression, anxiety, and pain will not fix you either. You can be stitched up, drugged up, and covered up, but if you want to be truly healed, you will have to do it yourself. Learning the basics is easy, and they lead to real change.

Thomas Edison said, "The doctor of the future will give no medicine but will interest his patients in the care of the human frame, in diet, and in the cause and prevention of disease." Thomas Edison, as we know, was ahead of his time, but that time has now come.

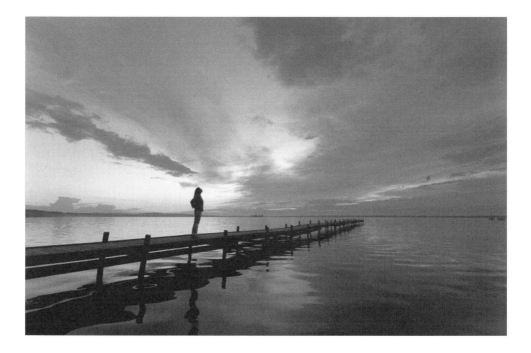

The Original Cause of physical illness often lies within the mind.

Chapter Two

The Link Between Body, Mind, and Spirit

OR

Why Your Thoughts and Feelings are Important

When Einstein proved that E = MC2 he was proving to the world that mass can convert into energy and back again. His discovery relates the world of things we touch to the world of energy we feel. We can touch things like our bodies but we can't really touch energy. We can't see it. Sometimes we can see the *results* of energy in a flash or a bang, but we rarely see what precedes energy or where it comes from.

As mass relates to energy, so energy relates to something even more invisible that, for simplicity's sake, I'll call thought. Ayurvedic doctors would categorize it as vata; Tibetan physicians refer to it as rlung. Others might call it spirit or essence. In our bodies we have properties of mass (or, if we're overweight, maybe too much mass), but we also have properties of energy. We experience our body's energy as warmth, digestive fire, or sometimes edginess. The lack of energy we call fatigue or even chronic fatigue. But our properties of thought and spirit are of an even higher order. They precede energy, causing it to exist and to move.

As difficult as it may be for science to test the physics of energy, it is virtually impossible for science to test the realm of thought, emotion, and intention. How do you quantify those qualities? Precisely because they can't be quantified scientifically, modern allopathic (Western) medicine has largely ignored the realm of spiritual health.

Holistic medical practitioners, however, do consider the realm of thought and feeling and acknowledge the power of love as possibly the greatest healer in the world.

Faith is another concept that most people choose to ignore simply because they don't quite know what to do with it. It seems old and outdated. But within the realm of thought, faith has substance. You can obtain it and develop it as a means for self-change and healing. Faith requires you to be emotionally open, receptive, and mentally alert. It is about right thoughts and right feeling, which equal right living. It exists in the realm of thought, feeling, sensation, will, love, and truth. It is not a theology but a philosophy of health and right living. Science and modern technology can certainly be very helpful, but don't forget your part in the greater workings of life. Making faith an active principle in your life is probably the best preventive medicine there is. It tends to keep you healthy.

The Holistic Approach to Healing

Modern Western medicine can do amazing things, particularly in emergency situations. Technological advancements in diagnosis and surgical procedures produce miracles everyday. In addition, we have a vast array of medications at our disposal to alleviate both emotional and physical pain. But the problem is that these medications rarely get to the root of or eradicate the cause of the pain.

Western medicine appears to have forgotten the ancient wisdom that tells us there are properties that can't be tested in double-blind, placebo-controlled studies. Nor has it caught up with the revolutionary discovery of quantum physics that time is malleable and energy is changeable. In a sense, Einstein began to prove what ancient practitioners knew intuitively, and traditional Western medicine is caught in a time warp between ancient wisdom and modern science.

Holistic physicians, on the other hand, who base their approach to medicine in part on the ancient traditional practices of India, China, and Tibet, understand and work with the principle that our thoughts and emotions can and do affect our physical health, and vice versa.

The Power of Positive Energy

The link between the mind and the body becomes rather obvious when we look at it on the level of sensation. How many times have you had a sugary drink and felt your energy increase and then precipitously decline? Have you noticed how sleepy everyone feels on Thanksgiving after feasting on a turkey rich in tryptophan? Does caffeine make you anxious or jittery? All these sensations can be explained simply in terms of biochemistry, but they also demonstrate unequivocally that what affects your body (mass) also affects your moods (energy).

Most of us have a particular level of energy with which we feel comfortable, and often, when our energy exceeds our comfort zone, we spill it out by telling jokes, engaging in some kind of physical activity, yawning, or even through negativity. One of the more negative ways we have of releasing emotional energy is to overeat, which is one example of how negative energy and excess energy can and do affect our physical health.

One of the most powerful tools there is for maximizing physical health is to increase your level of positive energy; you have that power within you right now, and in the following chapters I'll be providing you with information you need to put it to work in your life.

According to ancient teachings, when people die their energy becomes very high. That energy is released from the body and is transformed into another state of being, which I'll call spirit. This is one area in which, oddly enough, those who believe in the afterlife and those who understand the principles of quantum physics agree. Energy never dies; it is simply transformed. Mass becomes energy and, when we die, our energy goes into our spirit. And, similarly, negative energy can be transformed into positive energy.

To Transform Your Health, Change Your Thoughts

Although you may not be aware of it, not only your current thoughts and emotions but also the subconscious beliefs and emotional patterns created by your past are affecting you mentally and physically right now. You may think you can't help what you think, but you can. You may think you have no control over what you're not aware of, but you do. In this book I'll be providing techniques that will allow you not only to dump your current, negative thoughts and emotions but also to bring to consciousness and release hidden thoughts and feelings left over from your past so that they are no longer driving your behavior and limiting your potential for achieving optimum health.

Your body is linked to your thoughts and emotions. Holding onto negative, unproductive thoughts and feelings may be making you tired, angry, irritable, or tense. You can see those feelings if you look in the mirror. Tension shows up in your face; instead of open and relaxed, your expression will appear fixed and frozen. Rather than looking for a wrinkle cure by paralyzing your face with Botox, why not cure yourself of unnecessary wrinkles more naturally and permanently by getting rid of your tension and allowing your face to relax and be happy?

When you're unaware of the source of your tension or negative emotions and thoughts, you don't know how to release them in a positive way. Instead you might seek to relieve the stress they're causing with food. When you eat your body needs to focus its energy on digestion, and, as a result, thinking and emotions are dulled. Your worries become less stressful—at least temporarily. But then the vicious cycle continues.

If you're under constant stress you may be constantly overeating, which will result in your becoming overweight, over fat or ill, and the stress you put on your body will then create more stress for you mentally and emotionally. The purpose of this book is to set you on a different path, one that will allow your mental, physical, and emotional energies to work positively together instead of perpetuating a self-destructive cycle of negativity.

To get off the negative path you're on and get on the right one, I invite you to take the **10 steps to natural health** outlined in the following chapter.

The Spiritual Trinity of You

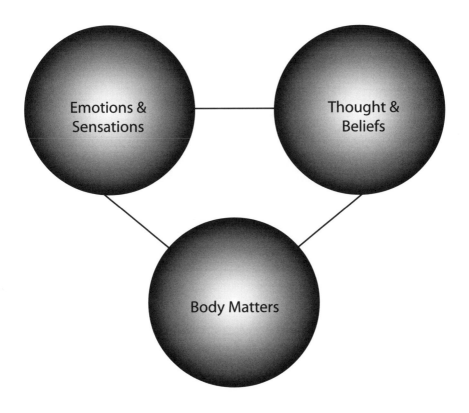

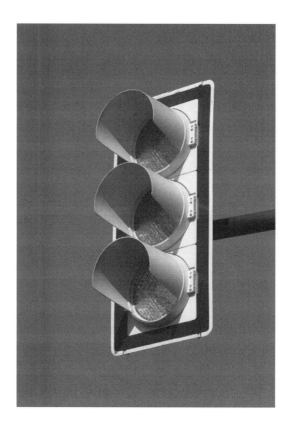

Stop

Become Aware

and

Start Living

Chapter Three

The 10 Steps to Natural Health

Apply the following steps to your own life one at a time in the order they are presented. Doing this may take a while and runs counter to modern society's desire for quick fixes and instant gratification—but that may have been what damaged your health in the first place. The point is that you *can* change. All you need to do is be willing to take charge of yourself and open yourself up to some new ideas. It's never too late to change unless you've told yourself that it is—and that, too, can change.

Step One
STOP Eating Unnatural Foods and START Eating Naturally

Eating naturally means consuming foods that are not chemically processed or genetically altered and that have evolved along with mankind. It means eating foods in their season and prepared naturally—that is, raw or cooked with fire or water. Even foods that are generally considered "healthy" can stress the body when we consume them unnaturally. For example, if we consume the equivalent of eight oranges in one glass of orange juice, which we swallow in thirty seconds, we are eating a natural food unnaturally. Doing that causes a rapid rise in blood sugar, which can stress the pancreas (leading to diabetes) or lead to excess storage of fat (causing obesity). Then, when our elevated blood sugar suddenly drops, we feel tired and want to consume more of the very food that caused our bad feeling in the first place.

The Toxic Effects of Scientific Advances

We now manufacture approximately 100,000 chemicals not naturally occurring in the air, water, or earth. In addition, there are chemicals that occur naturally in the earth and in plants but have never been part of the human food supply, and these too are now being introduced into the food production process. It may take another hundred years of scientific study to discover how each one of these chemicals affect the human body, which means that we probably won't be around to hear all the answers, but we already know that some of them are toxic. For example, potentially deadly, man-made polychlorobiphenyls, (used in insecticides, herbicides and other industrial uses), are everywhere in the environment. And roseotoxin, aflatoxin, rubratoxin and other naturally occurring toxins found in contaminated grains, are proliferating as a result of modern, large-scale production processes.

It's inevitable that some of these chemicals would find their way into the human body, but the problem is magnified when they are intentionally or accidentally introduced into our food supply. You could certainly wait to find out which of these 100,000 manmade chemicals are harmful, but wouldn't it be wiser to conclude that you ought to avoid them all as much as possible by following a diet that is in keeping with the natural evolutionary food chain? Small amounts of poisons (mercury for example), consumed daily for a lifetime, could degrade your health gradually until calamity occurs. You can use an air purifier or move to an area where the air is relatively clean. You can filter and test the purity of your drinking water. But the area where you have the most control is choosing the foods you eat.

What's Natural and What Isn't

When you're deciding what to put in your body, your first line of defense is to read the food labels on everything you buy. Simply assuming that any food manufactured for human consumption and approved by the Department of Agriculture is safe would be making a big mistake. It probably won't kill you right away, but that doesn't mean that it isn't going to damage your health over time. You would, therefore, be wise to take personal responsibility and not trust the government or food manufacturers to safeguard your health for you.

Unnatural foods—those with chemicals and additives and those that have been altered from their naturally occurring state in the manufacturing process—are those most likely to cause illness and/or chronic allergic reactions. Unnatural foods and unnaturally eaten foods have names like trans fatty acids, monosodium glutamate, oleo, margarine, and very long-chain fatty acids such as canola oil, and cottonseed oil. They're dyes and coloring agents called F, D, C # 4, and Red # 4. Sometimes they're just called artificial flavorings. Anything artificial is obviously not natural, and, therefore, you shouldn't be eating it.

There are, on the other hand chemicals that occur naturally but are not natural to the foods we eat. One of these is aluminum, which is found in the earth's crust but not in the evolutionary food chain. You may have heard about the dangers of aluminum leaching from cans, but did you know that it is also added to some of our foods? It's often found, for example, in pancake and waffle mixes, not to mention antacids. It's tragically ironic to think that the "medicine" we take to "cure" us of the reaction to something we shouldn't have eaten in the first place may actually be causing additional harm.

The body is a complex factory and needs some trace minerals, including gold and silver, to function. But it doesn't effectively differentiate between those it needs and those it doesn't, so whatever you eat will be absorbed—including mercury, which is known to be toxic.

Studies have shown a link between aluminum, along with very long-chain fatty acids, and Alzheimer's Disease. Although the specific role they might play has not yet been scientifically clarified, logic would suggest that until it is, we'd be better off avoiding them in our diet, along with other unnatural foods whose harmful effects may not yet have been discovered.

Another such danger lurks in fluoride, which is found naturally in green and black teas and is also an ingredient in most commercial toothpastes. Fluoride has been associated with hypothyroid problems, ADHD, Alzheimer's Disease, osteoporosis, arthritis, psychosis, kidney problems, headache, central nervous system problems, and memory problems, and works against beneficial antioxidants. We can certainly avoid drinking black and green teas, but fluoride does help to prevent tooth decay. To balance those benefits against the risks of ingesting too much, I personally don't drink black or green teas, and I read food labels to be sure they are not present in other foods I eat. I do brush my teeth morning and night with a fluoride toothpaste, but I rinse thoroughly and avoid swallowing the toothpaste. During the day, when I brush after eating, I use a non-fluoride ayurvedic toothpaste. My solution to the problem combines science and logic to arrive at a balance between risk and benefit that will be most beneficial to my health.

You Can't Change a Lifetime of Habits Overnight

In today's world, children, more often than not, start their day with orange juice, a Pop Tart covered in sugary syrup or butter, and a glass of chocolate milk. As an adult you may have coffee and a doughnut before rushing off to work, snack through lunch, rush home, have a glass of wine or a cocktail to relax, call out for pizza that is covered in cheese and acidic tomato paste, then drink more coffee to stay awake. Even as a "youthful" twenty-year-old, you may already have repeated patterns of poor eating, ill health, and consuming toxic foods up to 7000 times in your life. Chronic degradation and illness can occur even at a "young" age.

Stress at work increases stomach acid, which leads to ulcers and/or esophageal reflux, your thoughts become confused, creativity declines, and you can't wait to get home, where the stress manifests as family fights. Your natural happiness and sense of peace are eroded, and eating for pleasure becomes your primary coping mechanism. Does this pattern sound familiar?

The problem is then compounded when you "order out" or eat in restaurants on a regular basis. The fact is that if you don't prepare your own food, you don't know what's in it. And, more often than not, if you ask, the person who is serving you doesn't know either. I can assure you, however, that you'll be eating a lot more canola and cottonseed oil than good fats and essential fatty acids. This is particularly true if you're consuming inexpensive fast food. Inexpensive usually means industrial grade food.

You can change that pattern. You can decide to live better and stop harming yourself. But if you've been eating unnatural, contaminated, or incompatible foods since you were a small child, you may not be aware that angst, irritability, cramps, flatulence, mucous, constipation, and difficulty sleeping are not normal. You become used to feeling depressed, yelling at people, using sleep aids and other medications. And, everyone else seems to have similar problems! As a result, finding your way to better health may take a leap of faith because it is something you don't remember or may never have known.

It will also take time. It can take as much as a year to undo and correct the lifetime of harm you've been doing to your body, mind, and spirit. But with each new lifestyle and nutrition choice you make you will be taking one more step toward recovery. Every improvement on one level, such as nutrition, will create improvement on another level, such as mental clarity and willpower, and vice versa.

The Way to Natural Eating

Natural foods are grown without the use of chemicals and ripened in their season. To eat naturally is to follow a primarily vegetarian diet, perhaps with small amounts of lean meat. These foods should also be eaten in as close to their natural state as possible, which means raw, cooked in water or over fire, and on occasion in natural oils such as olive, sunflower, or sesame oil. And finally, you should be eating only when you are hungry, not because you think its mealtime, to be sociable, or as a means of self-soothing. Actual hunger originates from your abdomen as a feeling whereas false hunger originates from your mind as the result of anxiety or boredom.

As a species, we humans evolved eat a mainly vegetarian or plant-based diet. The dental patterns of our ancestors show them to have existed mainly on plant-based foods. And those animals they did consume were much leaner, healthier, and less contaminated than any farm-raised animal today. Therefore, a vegetarian diet is the preferred and safest course of human eating as long as you make sure it is supplemented with high quality vitamins and, on occasion, amino acids.

The primary reason to follow a mainly plant-based or vegetarian diet is one you're no doubt already aware of—high fat diets increase your risk for developing vascular plaque, which leads to arthrosclerosis, the number-one cause of death and physical disease in America. Vascular plaque is composed of fat, cholesterol, and mineral deposits that form inside the blood vessels, and cholesterol is found only in animal products. Anything that didn't walk on the earth, fly in the air, or swim in the sea does not contain dietary cholesterol.

Our bodies also manufacture cholesterol, which is a structural component of our cells' membranes and essential for sustaining life. The problems begin when we get too much of it from dietary sources. Stress, depression, and lack of exercise can also raise cholesterol levels. Natural cholesterol-lowering foods include evening primrose oil, cod liver oil, olive oil, lecithin, carnitine, fiber (found primarily in fruits and vegetables) oat bran, garlic, and vitamins C and E. All of these natural methods of lowering cholesterol are safer than taking synthetic statin drugs that can interfere with the liver's ability to eliminate toxins from the body and ultimately destroy it.

Sugar, while natural, is being consumed at the rate of about 175 pounds per person per year compared with an average of 15 pounds 50 years ago. This increasing sugar overload has led to an increase in metabolic syndrome (syndrome X) and Type 2 diabetes. Caffeine, while also natural, is being pumped into every health, weight loss, and sports drink possible as a way to "treat" the fatigue of sugar consumption and the stress of the western work place. Caffeine is a drug that adversely affects blood sugar, heart rhythms, anxiety, and insomnia among other symptoms of ill-health. Alcohol, while probably not harmful in very small amounts, is known to stress the liver, causing cirrhosis, and to impair responsible consciousness.

From a cultural point of view, these foods are both sign and symptom, cause and result of an overstressed society. The interconnectedness of body, mind, and emotions is clearly indicated by the increased consumption of sugar, caffeine, and alcohol, not only in America but by native populations throughout the world that are experiencing increased incidences of diabetes and hypertension as a result of their increased exposure to the western diet.

"Health" Foods to Avoid

Many of you are no doubt already aware that some foods are "healthier" than others. In truth, it would be almost impossible to avoid hearing the health claims being made for certain foods. Unfortunately, however, many of these claims don't tell you the whole story. There are, in fact, three so-called health foods that actually could be making you sick. They are canola oil, seafood, and unfermented soy.

Canola oil is an artificially produced, genetically modified oil derived from the inedible and very toxic rapeseed oil. It contains glycosides (organic compounds that affect the heart) and extra long chain fatty acids, which are unnatural to the body and have been associated with diseases that destroy the myelin sheath coating the nervous system structures.

Seafood has, to a large degree, been contaminated with mercury, which has been associated with chronic fatigue and birth defects. Although tuna is the fish most associated with mercury, virtually any seafood can contain this contaminant. Fish caught in the waters off the Pacific Northwest and Alaska appear to contain the least. Farm raised fish tend to contain other toxins called polychlorobiphenyls, which have been associated with cancer, endocrine disorders, and sterility.

Unfermented soy contains hemagglutins and phytoestrogens. Hemagglutins cause blood cells to clump, leading to the slowing or blockage of circulation to the capillaries. Phytoestrogens are plant-based estrogens that mimic human estrogens, causing a feminine shift in the endocrine balance, which may have feminizing effects, particularly on still-developing boys and may be associated with erectile dysfunction and/or impotence in men. Fermentation removes these toxic components, and throughout history native cultures have consumed *fermented* soy. Unfermented soy is a recent phenomenon created by the health-food industry.

Indulge in Good Health

If you eat to pamper yourself, why not pamper yourself by preparing your own meals with ingredients you have chosen because you know they are healthy and soothing to your body as well as your mind and your emotions.

STOP Taking Inexpensive Nutritional Products and START Taking a High Quality Vitamin, Mineral, Essential Fatty Acid and Natural Vitamin E Supplement

If you raise all your own food in ground that is fertile and has never been contaminated by fertilizers, pesticides, herbicides, insecticides, mining, or manufacturing, and if you know your water supply is equally uncontaminated, you can skip this chapter. If, on the other hand, you're like the remaining 99.9 percent of us who buy our food from commercial sources, you need to be taking high quality nutritional supplements. Unfortunately, commercial farmers are not paid for the quality but for the quantity of food they produce, which means that most of what we eat is often deficient in the nutrients that naturally produced food would contain. Commercial produce is often harvested before it's fully ripe and may, therefore, be nutrient deficient. And overproduced soil may be lacking in trace minerals such as manganese, molybdenum, boron, vanadium, and zinc, which will also then be lacking in the foods grown in that soil. A deficiency of any one of these minerals can make you more susceptible to illness or infection. Your body, for example, needs zinc in order to fight bacterial infections.

Some experts believe that up to 85 percent of the population is deficient in vitamin D. And although organic food is supposed to be uncontaminated and more nutritious, there are various levels of standards that permit purveyors to use the term "organic" on their labels even when the products may not be that pure. What all this means is that even when you begin to eat naturally, you should be supplementing your diet with high quality products.

What You Should Know about the Quality of Your Supplements

If you've been buying your supplements in a grocery or drug store, chances are that you've not been getting what you think you paid for. Not only can't you be sure that what is written on the label is actually in the product, you also have to be concerned about what's *not* on the label. There are recent efforts for supplement manufacturers to produce their goods with a (GMP) "good manufacturing process" standard of approval. Time will show whether this quality control is really helpful.

If the manufacturer is cutting corners or driven only by profit, the quantity of a nutrient that is actually contained in the product may be significantly smaller than that listed on the label. In addition, cheaper supplements may be made with all kinds of unnatural fillers, binders, lubricating agents and colorings that could actually be harming your body.

Fillers and preservatives are added to increase volume and prevent deterioration. The problem is that some of these fillers and preservatives, such as lactose, sodium benzoate, BHA, BHT, and hydrogenated oils, can trigger allergic reactions.

Coloring agents, which are often synthetically derived, serve no purpose at all except to make the supplement look more attractive so that you will be more likely to buy it. The fact is that most additives, fillers, and binders do not have to be listed on the label.

Obtaining your supplements from a trustworthy, high quality manufacturer will minimize your risk of getting these chemicals along with your vitamins and minerals. I also recommend that you stop taking all nutritional products for up to a week before adding a high quality product so that you are able to get a "read" on what your natural baseline of health actually feels like.

How Can You Tell Whether It's High Quality?

One way of determining the quality of your vitamins is to check the vitamin E content and see if the label says "d" tocopherols or "dl" tocopherols. Vitamin E is made up of a group of closely related fat-soluble alcohols called tocopherols. "D" tocopherols are natural; "l" tocopherols are synthetic. Synthetic vitamin E is made with equal parts "d" and "l" tocopherols, but the human body is able to metabolize only the natural "d" tocopherols, so half of what you're getting in synthetic vitamin E your body is unable to use. Although there's no scientific evidence to indicate that synthetic tocopherols are harmful, it would seem logical to avoid them if possible, and, in any case, why would you want to pay for a product that is only half useful to your body? Beyond that, however, science has identified several forms of naturally occurring tocopherols, called alpha, gamma, and delta, and there may be more not yet identified. Good supplements will contain a combination of these and not just the most common "d alpha" form. So do check the label to be sure you're getting the best.

When it comes to minerals, how they are combined in the capsule determines how much of what you're taking is absorbed and how much simply goes through your body untouched. Magnesium citrate is better absorbed than magnesium oxide, for example. And those that say they are chelated or that they're bound with aspartate, citrate, and piccolinate are generally the healthiest.

Some nutrients, such as coenzyme Q10, folate, and B12/biotin deteriorate quickly, and the form they are in (crystalline, water-soluble, or oil soluble) also affects how much the body can absorb; it's important to choose forms of these nutrients that are most bio-absorbable and free from degradation. How they are bound to other molecules affects how much the body can actually absorb. Cheaper vitamin companies tend to use cheap products that do not allow the essential nutrients to be released and absorbed into the body. So, for example, a label might say the product contains 100mg of a particular vitamin but only 10% of that amount may actually be released and absorbed into the body when you swallow it.

Capsules, Liquids, Powders, or Pills—Which Form is Best?

Anything that comes in pill form—as opposed to capsules, liquids, or bulk powders—requires artificial binders to hold it together. Manufacturers also use lubricants like magnesium stearate, stearic acid, ascorbyl palmitate, and canola oil to make the pills go through the machinery.

These products do nothing for your health and wind up coating the pills with lubricating material that can not only interfere with their absorption but could also be introducing more harmful chemicals into your body. Therefore, I recommend that you take supplements only in capsule, liquid, or powder form, none of which require the use of these additives in their manufacture.

Which Supplements and Why

Compared to herbs (which I'll be discussing in the next step) and prescription drugs, nutritional supplements are the safest class of healing products you can take. There are, however, a few caveats.

Fat soluble vitamins like A and D can be stored in excess and do damage to your liver and kidneys respectively. Vitamin K can interfere with Coumadin, which is commonly prescribed as a blood thinner. So you should consult a holistic doctor or a nutritionist if you have any doubts or are taking other medications.

That said, however, the dearth of nutrients in so many commercially grown foods, and the pesticides, herbicides, and insecticides used to produce them, mean that we all need to be taking supplemental natural vitamins E and C as well as zinc and selenium to protect us from the harm caused by oxidants, free-radicals, and carcinogens in the body.

Given the chemical assault on the body most of us experience every day, I believe that taking natural vitamin E is one of the most important steps we can take to protect ourselves. Even some scientific studies of patients with cancer, heart attacks, stroke, and other illnesses are beginning to confirm the improved survival rates that result from taking vitamin E. (1000 IU mixed natural vitamin E is considered a safe dose)

That said, however, there are always limits to how much is too much, and science is still testing those limits. Everything known—including water—can be lethal if you ingest enough of it. So do your own research and, most of all, take a break from every product every so often to allow your body time to find its own balance.

Other natural nutrients that can provide anti-oxidants and anti-cancer protection include grapeseed extract (proanthocyanidins), lycopene (tomato), inositol, curcumin (turmeric), plant oxidants, bilberry extract, milk thistle extract, quercetin, alpha-lipoic acid, and red clover. You may decide to take these one at a time for a week to boost your immune system on the cellular level, but you should first consult a holistic doctor because even too many helpful chemicals can overwhelm your body.

Anyone who is anemic and all women who are menstruating should also take an iron supplement. Iron can, however, upset your stomach, so you'll need to read the label to determine the form in which it is given. Iron can be ferrous, ferric iron citrate, and iron picolinate, the last of which is usually the best absorbed and least irritating to the stomach.

Women should also be taking extra calcium and magnesium, along with vitamin D3 to protect against bone loss. Look for supplements that contain a combination of these three products.

Essential Fatty Acids (EFAs) are, as the name implies, essential to your body. What you may not realize, however, is that the term "essential" means that the body can not manufacture them and that we, therefore, need to get them from food or from supplements. The two essential fatty acids are omega 3 and omega 6 from which your body then makes other fatty acids.

Your nerves are 80 percent fat, the brain is 60 percent fat, and every cell in your body is protected and lined by fatty acids, as are the mitochondria, or power sources, within the cells. Artificial and unnatural fatty acids have for years been added to virtually all commercial foods, so, in addition to eliminating the unnatural fats, you need to re-supply your body with natural EFAs. Omega 3s are found in refined fish oil and flaxseed oil and omega 6s are in primrose oil and blackcurrant oil. According to the most scientific studies, you need them in a ratio of 4 parts omega 3, to 1 part omega 6.

Step Three

STOP Taking Herbal Medications Incorrectly

If you've been concerned about taking too many prescription medications you may have been taking herbs because you believe that at best they will improve your health and at worst they won't cause any harm. The trouble is that you may have been taking them on a prolonged ongoing basis, and that's not the way herbs are meant to be used.

While it's certainly true that herbs are generally safer than prescription medications, if you're taking anywhere from ten to thirty herbs every day for years on end, that is not natural. Herbs are meant to provide *temporary* relief and to balance your health. They need to be metabolized, detoxified, and excreted from the body like any other chemical, and taken long-term they can overwhelm your detoxifying systems including the liver, kidneys, skin, lungs, and bowel.

They can have side effects just like prescription medications, and when that happens, you could wind up dealing with the side effects by taking even more herbs or even a prescription product. I once had a patient who asked me to evaluate his health situation who had been taking between ten and thirty different herbs every day for years and clearly was overwhelming his detoxification system. In addition to advising that he get a chest X-ray and a CT head scan for his particular concerns, I advised him to stop all his herbs for two weeks and then begin taking only those which he thought he really needed. Sadly, he never really did all that I suggested, and he died a year and a half later from lung cancer that had metastasized to his brain. We'll never know what exactly caused his cancer, but to me it seemed clear that his massive over consumption of herbs had created a chemical insult to his body.

Although they have been used for centuries by indigenous cultures throughout the world, herbs have also been misused. Marijuana, cocaine, alcohol, caffeine, chocolate, tobacco, and opium have all been considered herbs at one time, and all have been misused. And the misuse of each one of these substances has caused mental, emotional, and physical decline.

46

You need to use herbs responsibly, just as you would any other substance you put in your body.

They ought to be remedies for temporary problems, no addictive lifestyle crutches for daily coping. If you have any doubt about the proper use of any one herb or herbs in general, you should check with an herbalist or a holistic or naturopathic medical doctor.

Children and pregnant women are particularly limited in the kinds of herbs they can take safely. Belladonna, bloodroot, and mistletoe are particularly dangerous, but any herb used long enough or in combination with a prescription medication can be harmful. Do not assume because they are herbs they are safe.

The Right Way to do It

In traditional Chinese, ayurvedic, and Tibetan medicine specific combinations of herbs are used for a period of two to three months to balance the system. In the simplest of terms, Chinese medicine refers to balancing "chi" or the flow of energy—wet with dry, hot with cold—the five elements (wood, fire, earth, metal, and water), and yin with yang (the complementary life forces). Ayurvedic (or Tibetan) medicine refers to vata (rlung), pitta (beygen), and kapha (phlegm). Creating this balance occurs gradually, which is why herbs are generally prescribed for a period of two to three months, along with lifestyle and dietary changes. At the end of those few months, however, the herbs are stopped and naturally occurring nutritional, lifestyle, mental, and emotional changes are expected to continue keeping your body healthy and protected.

Herbs can also be taken singly for a particular complaint. When taken this way the herb has a strong effect on the body, but it is generally used for less than two weeks.

Modern science has been able to validate the chemical effect of herbs on our bodies, but because we don't yet know exactly how herbs work, medical science has been reluctant to support them fully. Pharmaceutical testing is normally done on one chemical at a time, but the nature of herbs is that they work in combination with one another and different combinations create different, naturally occurring chemical effects. In addition, a single herb may contain 100 bioactive molecules, which means that the standard method of altering one variable at a time cannot be applied to their testing. This makes them difficult to test scientifically, but one would hope that with more experimentation and the integration of health science with health philosophy, this reluctance to embrace the use of herbs will diminish. Many prescription medications are, in fact, derived from naturally occurring plant products.

Step Four

STOP or Reduce Your Prescription Drug Use

Traditional MD (allopathic) and DO (osteopathic) doctors are accustomed to prescribing medications to treat your ills, but rarely do they consider taking a patient *off* medication when a problem arises. In fact, part of every doctor's medical training, including my own, is learning how to prescribe medications while nutrition education is minimal at best.

The truth is, however, that prescription medications are vastly overused in modern medicine. In fact, health management as it is traditionally practiced depends primarily upon the management of medications. These medications may then cause side effects, and rather than telling you to reduce the dosage or stop taking the drug altogether, doctors generally prescribe yet another medication to counteract the side effects of the one you're already taking. Nor do they think of taking you off a medication that may no longer be needed. Logically, you can see how you might wind up taking multiple drugs, many of them simply to manage the symptoms caused by others that were previously prescribed.

Although doctors know that prescription medications can and do have side effects, there are thousands of drugs with hundreds of thousands of side effects, including some we're not even aware. Cholesterol lowering medications (statins), for example, can deplete coenzyme Q10 and damage the liver, and hydrochlorothiazide (HCTZ), a diuretic used to lower blood pressure, can raise levels of LDL (bad) cholesterol and triglycerides. In one particularly dramatic example of dangerous side effects, a patient of mine had been prescribed the blood-thinner Coumadin, the "standard of care" medication for treating atrial fibrillation and leg clots. Subsequently she developed a condition known as idiopathic thrombocytopenia purpura, which means that for reasons unknown (i.e., idiopathic) her body had stopped making blood platelets. Platelets aid the clotting process and prevent you from bleeding to death. You should have approximately 200,000 per cc (cubic centimeter) of blood; this woman's had dropped to less than 5, which meant she was bleeding to death. She was quickly given a replacement of the lost platelets as a temporary measure and taken off the Coumadin. Ironically, Coumadin is not known to cause a decrease in platelet production, but four other medications she was also taking listed thrombocytopenia as a possible side effect. However, neither her primary care physician nor the specialist she was seeing for her potentially fatal blood disorder thought to look up the potential side effects of these medications in the *Physician's Desk Reference (PDR)*, a standard reference tool on every doctor's desk. When that was done, she was able to get to the root of her bleeding problem and find safer, more natural alternatives for treating her other health issues. After several hospitalizations and specialized treatment for her bleeding disorder, she was taken off her previous medications and her platelets returned to normal levels.

In addition to their potentially dangerous side effects and interactions, most medicines are being prescribed in far higher doses than are necessary. The aim should be to take as low a dose as possible to achieve the effect you seek both to minimize side effects and because all drugs are chemicals that can stress and overload the detoxification organs in your body. The extra work your body must do to accommodate these medications can actually weaken rather than increase your ability to fight off disease. And, according to a study conducted by Bruce

Pomeranz M.D., PH.D., of the University of Toronto and published in the distinguished *Journal of the American Medical Association (JAMA)*, between one in four and one in six deaths result from prescription drug problems—the wrong prescription, side effects from the medication, or improper use of the medication prescribed.

That said, prescription drugs are certainly beneficial for people who are hypertensive, diabetic, or who have cardiac problems. Many other ailments, however, are, in my opinion, either wrongly or too quickly treated with prescription medications when they would be better and more safely alleviated through nutritional and/or lifestyle changes or with counseling. Mood and mind affecting drugs that mask the symptoms rather than uncovering and correcting the causes are particularly overused for sleep problems, depression, chronic pain, and personality disorders.

Medications for heartburn and stomach distress (such as "the little purple pill" called Nexium) are also overused, as are cholesterol lowering statin drugs that can damage the liver. Both gastrointestinal distress and elevated cholesterol can often be improved with dietary changes—such as eating more plant-based foods, more fiber, more omega 3 fatty acids, less dairy, and fewer egg yolks—as well as with more natural herbal products and increased exercise. If you are willing to do something more natural, you can often come off prescription medication. Do this with the advice and supervision of a doctor.

It's Not Necessarily All the Doctor's Fault

I said earlier that Coumadin is considered the "standard of care" for treating atrial fibrillation. That term has, unfortunately, become a legal term dangling over the doctor's head like the sword of Damocles, and, in my opinion, doing more harm than good. Once it has been decided, as the result of studies done by academics or even pharmaceutical companies, that a particular protocol or medication is the best course of treatment for a particular health problem, that protocol or medication becomes the "standard of care" that all doctors are expected to follow if they don't want to risk being sued for malpractice. Clearly, this allows very little room for individualized care or for doctors to use their own judgment.

Add to those constraints the pressure put upon medical practitioners by the managed care system to treat as many people as possible in the shortest possible time for the least amount of money, not to mention the hours they must devote to the reams of paperwork generated by the system, and it's easy to understand why doctors would be anxious to find the medication that would treat the problem as simply and quickly as possible.

Generally that translates into not only prescribing too many medications but also the often unnecessarily high doses recommended by the manufacturer, because using less might take longer and would also require figuring out on a patient-by-patient basis how little is enough but not too much.

If you think you're receiving too high a dose of a particular medication, ask your doctor if it would be possible to lower it, at least on a trial basis.

Do Take Responsibility, but Don't Try to Do this on Your Own

Never lower a prescribed dose or discontinue a medication without consulting your doctor. Narcotics, anti-depressants, and blood pressure medications, among others, must be tapered off slowly and should be adjusted only with a doctor's supervision.

In many cases, however, you may no longer need a medication you've been taking, or you may not need to be taking as much of it. If you've been on medication for diabetes, for example, you may no longer need it if you've changed your diet and lost weight. The same may be true for blood pressure medication when you begin to take magnesium and start an exercise program such as walking.

Still, many doctors will be taken aback if you ask to reduce the dose or discontinue a medication, and they may be resistant. Standard medical thinking, after all, is that once you start taking a medication (unless it is an antibiotic or a short-term pain killer) you will probably be on it for the rest of your life.

Not only that, but once you leave his office after your annual or semi-annual visit, your doctor virtually never reviews your chart until the next time you appear or call. In fact, he probably doesn't even think about you. He certainly won't be thinking, hmm, Jane Doe has been taking this medication for three (or six or nine) months; maybe we should call her up and ask her to come in to see if she still needs it or if we should lower the dose. In fact, even when you do come in for a routine check up, unless something seems to be going wrong, he probably won't think about changing the medications you're taking. If, for instance, you've been taking medication to lower your blood pressure, the doctor will certainly check your pressure, but if it's normal he won't consider whether or not you could lower the dose or change the medication.

You, the patient, are the one who will have to make that suggestion. You are, after all, the person ultimately responsible for your own health.

Step Five

STOP Dieting—Diets are Counterproductive

Notice that I'm not saying you should stop losing weight. As I discussed in Chapter One, obesity is an illness that has reached epidemic proportions in America. What I am saying is that dieting never works in the long term and is, in fact, comparable to taking antidepressant medication in that it alleviates the symptoms (at least temporarily) without ever getting to the root of what caused you to become overweight in the first place.

One of the reasons I say that dieting is counterproductive is that it causes you to think about food all the time. Those thoughts take up residence in your subconscious, and as soon as you stop dieting, the first thing you do is eat all the food you've been thinking about not eating.

When that happens you are reinforcing the negative self-thoughts that were responsible for your overeating in the first place and diminishing the willpower and confidence you need to change those thoughts and make the nutritional and lifestyle changes that will lead to your losing the weight naturally and permanently.

So, if you need to lose weight, the last thing you should be thinking about is food. You should be walking, running, or doing some form of exercise like yoga to alleviate the stress in your life that probably led you to overeat in the first place.

Diets are All About Food

Diets have come and gone over the years. You may have tried or at least heard about many of them. Each one has contributed something to our knowledge of the relationship between nutrition and health, but none of them adequately addresses the mental and emotional issues related to health and obesity.

In the 1950s Nathan Pritikin, a layman with an engineering background, introduced the concept of drastically reducing the amount of meat and fat in our diet while simultaneously increasing our intake of fiber. Pritikin's contribution set the standard for heart-healthy diets in the next half century, but he didn't understand the need for healthy dietary fats such as omega 3 essential fatty acids, and he inadvertently created the market for any number of artificially engineered "low fat" and "low calorie" foods including artificial sweeteners that may actually be undermining the healthy principles he embraced.

Then, in the mid-eighties, Dr. Dean Ornish built upon what Pritikin had started with *Dr. Dean Ornish's Program for Reversing Heart Disease.* Dr. Ornish brought all the medical credentials and scientific research Pritikin lacked to his program for reversing coronary artery disease without drugs or surgery. Like Pritikin's, his diet was extremely low in fat and calories, but it did not eliminate sugar, which has proved to be the one food possibly most responsible for much of our ill health. Ornish did, however, emphasize lifestyle changes to go along with his diet, and more recently he has begun to recommend yoga and meditation for relieving stress.

Whatever their shortcomings, however, these two low-fat pioneers have made a significant contribution by letting millions of people know how reducing our fat intake can reduce the risk for both heart disease and cancer.

Since then we've also had *The Mediterranean Diet,* Dr. Phil McGraw's *The Ultimate Weight Solution, The Zone,* and most recently *The South Beach Diet.* Each one, and many others like them, have taught us something about nutrition but none has had the far-reaching impact of *Dr. Atkins' Diet Revolution.*

As far back as 1980, Dr. Robert Atkins was going against the low-fat tide by recommending a diet that allowed you to eat as much protein and fat as you wanted but virtually no carbohydrates at all—including fruits and vegetables. Since then, the "new" Atkins diet has revised these recommendations to include 20 grams of carbs and no more than 20% of calories from fat.

When you follow it religiously, Atkins's diet does cause weight-loss because it takes advantage of the biophysical pathways through which we metabolize nutrients. Our bodies metabolize all carbohydrates as sugar, and if you eat more of them than you burn you will store the extra sugar as fat. If you stop eating carbohydrates, however, your body will go into reverse and start to burn fat. To the degree that Dr. Atkins recognized how much sugar most Americans were eating and how much that has contributed to the obesity epidemic in this country he was certainly on the mark.

Protein has low caloric value and tends to be metabolized for energy or to build muscle tissue. Fats also tend to get broken down into energy and are less likely than carbohydrates to be stored as fat. That might seem counterintuitive but it is actually how the body works.

So what's the problem? Well, for one thing, too much protein can stress the kidneys by creating an excess of caustic breakdown products like urea and ammonia. High protein diets have also been linked to stress on the liver and adrenal glands, and they may be responsible for polypeptide absorption from the bowel that can lead to chronic allergies.

Body-builders believe they must eat large quantities of protein in order to build muscle, but two of the strongest, most muscular animals on earth are the gorilla and the bull, both of which are vegetarian. Even infants, during the most significant growth period of human life, consume breast milk, which is less than 2 percent protein.

Additionally, the relatively high fat consumption of Atkins's and other low carb diets means that you're taking in a lot of calories (1 gram of fat has twice as many calories as either 1 gram of protein or 1 gram of carbohydrate), which need to be burned off somehow. And the additional fat can also stress the liver and gallbladder. High fat has also been linked to high levels of lipoprotein and fat in the blood, which are, in turn, linked to increased risk for atherosclerosis, heart attack, and stroke.

And then there's the psychological problem of never eating another piece of pizza, another bowl of pasta, or another potato for the rest of your life. If you haven't gotten to the root of your emotional issues with food to begin with, there will certainly be a high-carb binge some time in your future.

Seek Freedom, Not Restriction

While all the most popular diets—Atkins's in particular—emphasize what you *can* eat, they all work by restricting your choices. They are really about what you *can't* eat. That is, after all, what you're thinking about whenever you decide to "go on a diet." And because it's about restriction, it puts you in a negative mind-frame, and you know starting out that you're not going to stick with it forever. It's something you plan to do temporarily, until you reach your goal weight or fit into your "skinny jeans." And then what happens?

As I've been saying all along, unless you deal with the mental and emotional issues that have caused and contributed to your weight gain, you're condemning yourself to a lifetime of on-again-off-again yo-yo dieting that will ultimately cause even more damage to your health.

I don't believe in dieting or calorie-counting, which only increase your preoccupation with food. I prefer to live more freely and "wholly." A diet is something you "have" to do—for now; a lifestyle change, on the other hand, can permanently and happily affect your weight and your life. Of course, you do need to educate yourself about food and nutrition in order to make informed decisions, but it can be fun, and making new discoveries will open up a whole new world of edible and livable possibilities.

Step Six

STOP Eating Incompatible Foods

Incompatible foods are those that, for reasons unique to your particular body, are not properly digested and absorbed and may, therefore, be causing immunologic, or what are generally thought of as allergic reactions. If you eat them you may experience one or more of a whole host of symptoms including diarrhea or constipation, belching, passing gas, smelly stool, bloating, anxiety, irritability, depression, fatigue, hyperactivity, swollen eyes, cravings, weight gain, joint pain, coughing, sore throat, mucous, stuffy or runny nose, headache, insomnia, rash, itching, acne, asthma, forgetfulness, lack of focus, or frequent illness.

While none of these reactions is as immediately life-threatening as the anaphylactic type of allergic reaction some people have to a bee sting or to peanuts, for example, and they may, therefore, seem more annoying than alarming, they are really just the tip of the iceberg—the most obvious manifestations of more serious damage being done inside your body. A lifetime of eating incompatible foods can make you ill by stimulating your immune system to basically attack itself. If you continuously eat foods that are incompatible with your body, you can develop full-blown arthritis, seizures, ADHD, and obesity down the road. In my opinion, Western science has not yet recognized the full potential of the damage that eating incompatible foods can do to organs and vessels.

By discovering your own food incompatibilities, and cutting those foods out of your diet, you will live better, happier, healthier, and younger.

The Difference Between Immediate and Delayed Allergic Reactions
Your body has many kinds of immunoglobins or antibodies—IgG, IgM, IgE, and IgA—that are released into the bloodstream in response to an infection or an allergen. The quick-response, quick rash, can't breath, can't swallow type of allergic reaction is triggered only by the release of the IgE immunoglobulin. All of the remaining types create a slower more subtle response to other allergens, which generally result from eating incompatible foods on an ongoing basis. One of the most common and widely recognized of these types of sensitivities is to gluten, which is a chemical found in most grains. Even if you are not initially sensitive

to a particular food, however, eating it over and over again can cause a sensitivity to develop or to worsen.

What happens is that your body can't process the food properly; it isn't fully digested. As time goes on, if you continue to eat these foods, you'll be putting more and more strain on your digestive system, so your symptoms will become increasingly severe. Besides a cellular level of dysfunction, you may then begin to experience an organ level of dysfunction. That's one of the reasons I recommend that you eat foods according to their season, so that your body will have time to recover from the effects of your continually eating any one particular food.

You also need to eat a combination of acidic and alkaline foods to keep your body in balance; however, alkaline foods are generally thought to be more healthy for your body on a ph level. (See the Appendix for a list of acidic and alkaline foods.)

There are few companies that do reliable testing for immunologic responses. One that I sometimes recommend for patients who are experiencing a major illness is Immuno Laboratories. You can also do an elimination diet to discover which foods may be causing your particular reactions, but your first line of defense should be simply paying attention to your body and understanding that if you have any of the symptoms mentioned above on a regular basis, that is *not normal*. The foods your body reacts to as poison may, however, be perfectly healthy for somebody else. Ultimately, your inability to properly digest particular foods may be related to your unique genetic code and genetic history.

Start by eliminating the foods that are known to be most allergenic, such as cow dairy products and gluten (wheat products). (For a list of the most allergenic and hypoallergenic foods see the Appendix.) Adding one food at a time back to a hypoallergenic diet should enable you to determine if that food is giving you unwanted symptoms. Once you've identified an incompatible food, eliminate it entirely for at least three months to allow your body to recover. After that, you may be able to eat it from time to time with minimal insult to your body.

Why Eliminating Incompatible Foods is So Important

As I've said, the symptoms you may be experiencing are only the tip of the iceberg. The conflict that's going on inside your body can lead not only to outright illness but also to mental and emotional disturbances such as anxiety and brain fog or an inability to focus.

Some foods, such as sugar and caffeine, when eaten to excess, can actually become addictive. When you eliminate these foods, you will actually go through a period of withdrawal and may feel worse before you begin to feel better. However, the reward of regaining full control of your physical, emotional, and mental health is always worth the temporary discomfort. Eliminating incompatible foods from your unique body will give you the gift of long-term health.

Step Seven

START Walking—START Exercising

I'm not asking you to become a body-builder or an Olympic athlete, but luckily almost everyone can walk. You can do it virtually anywhere, and you don't need any special equipment beyond a pair of good walking shoes. Start with going one block if that's all you can do and build up gradually from there—walking faster, walking farther, walking more often. Walk in the park or the country on weekends; walk to work during the week. In addition to increasing your levels of HDL (good, heart healthy) cholesterol, walking provides fresh air to your lungs and stimulates the bowel. Walking allows your mind to slow down, relax, and engage in the kind of creative activity you don't always have time for when you're rushing from place and one activity to the next. It is a gentle way to start your day that can leave you in a healthy, peaceful frame of mind as you go about your regular activities. It's also a good de-stressor for the end of the day to walk and relax.

If you have any special health concern you should, of course, consult your doctor before you begin any kind of new exercise. And if you experience chest pain, shortness of breath, nausea, sudden sweatiness, light-headedness, or pain in your arms, back, or neck, you need to stop and seek medical attention. With those few caveats, however, walking is an activity that's available to just about everyone.

Beyond walking, however, I recommend that you also begin

a more formal exercise program that involves flexibility, aerobic, and strength training. Physical activity has more to do with achieving and maintaining health and proper body weight than all the food facts known.

The Three Elements of Proper Exercise

Flexibility: Before you begin any form of exercise you need to stretch and elongate your spine and your muscles. If you don't do that you will be working with short, tight muscles that are less powerful and less flexible. Yoga is a particularly useful form of exercise for developing flexibility.

Aerobic Exercise: Aerobics strengthen your heart and lungs by increasing your heart rate. Increasing your heart rate and breathing vigorously for 15 to 20 minutes at a time stimulates the lungs and blood vessels to flex and pump blood and oxygen more efficiently. I suggest some kind of aerobic exercise—which could be bicycling, running, rowing, or any other activity that emphasizes breathing—3 times a week. If you can't do 15 minutes, do what feels right for you and try to build up gradually.

Strength Training: Strength training or muscle resistance training is what most people think of as weight lifting. The weight doesn't have to be very heavy, but the resistance stimulates muscle growth and helps to increase bone density. For increasing general health you can do either more repetitions with less weight or fewer repetitions with more weight.

If you can't walk for any reason, try an alternative exercise such as swimming, which is easier on the joints. If you enjoy competitive sports, try tennis. Yoga, as I've said, helps to increase flexibility and can also provide a sense of spirituality. Exercising with a partner can help you to stay motivated on days when you'd rather stay in bed.

Whatever exercise you do, however, warm up slowly. Touch your legs, arms, and torso with your hands to coordinate your proprio-receptors—the joint and muscle receptors that provide information to your brain about limb position and movement as well as muscle length and tension—with your cerebellum, eyes, and hands. The proprio-receptors are one of the three balancing systems you need to stay upright; the other two are the eyes and the cerebellum/ears. Touching re-coordinates those systems to prepare for action.

Start any exercise at whatever level is comfortable for you and increase gradually. Set up a schedule that works for you, and try to exercise at the same time every day. By doing that your body will begin to prepare for you to "perform" at that time. And, finally, make sure you have the right kind of equipment and are using it properly. If you are walking or running, be sure to have a good pair of running shoes. To make sure that you're exercising right, it would be wise to consult a good trainer.

Why Exercise is Important

In addition to burning calories, improving flexibility, and reducing your risk for pulmonary and cardiovascular disease, exercise releases hormones that have positive effects both physically and mentally. If you have high blood pressure and are taking medication, you may find that with exercise and weight loss your need for medication will decrease. Medication for sleep, anxiety, stress, and even diabetes can sometimes be eliminated with the benefits of exercise.

Exercise stimulates the release of human growth hormone, which helps to increase muscle mass, revitalize organs, lower blood pressure, and decrease cholesterol and triglycerides in the blood.

Exercise also stimulates the release of endorphins, the "feel good" hormones that improve your mood and your ability to think clearly. Many people think of exercise as "work," but I would suggest that you think of it as freeing. It will free you to enjoy food more and to be healthier in every way. Always exercise in a positive state of mind.

Step Eight

START to Reconsider Your Lifestyle

Your lifestyle is an all-encompassing circle of holistic health that both results from and affects the choices you make, consciously or unconsciously, about how you interact with your environment. It both affects and is affected by your physical, mental, and emotional health. Taking the time to assess and reconsider your lifestyle can allow you to see where your stressors are coming from and how you react to them.

Start by asking yourself the following questions:

1 Am I happy?

2 Am I rested?

3 Do I have pleasure in my life?

4 Do I have time to devote to my family?

5 Am I overweight?

6 Am I motivated to do any one particular thing?

Once you've answered those questions you can start to be more specific so that your answers are even more helpful. It's usually easiest to start by re-examining a single day. Ask yourself:

1 Did I wake up relaxed or in a hurry?

2 Did I have a stressful day?

3 Did I have a conflict today, if so, why?

4 Did I live my life today with appreciation for true beauty and the positive things in my life?

5 What did I do for fun today?

6 What was the most fun thing I did today?

7 Why was it fun?

How Stressed Are You?

Chronic tension and stress may be the leading causes of chronic health problems. Stress is an indication that we don't have confidence or faith that "things will work out."

Do you need coffee to get you going in the morning? Coffee is a stimulant that can cause high blood pressure and destabilize blood sugar levels.

Do you have time for a five-minute stretch and a walk in the morning or are you rushing from the moment you get up? In nature you would have to walk to find food and water in the morning.

When you look in the mirror in the morning, is your face smooth and relaxed or already pinched and wrinkled from anticipated stress?

Do you feel pressured and rushed to complete your obligations throughout the day?

Do you have too much on your plate, causing you to compensate by putting too much on your dinner plate?

When you get home in the evening, do you have time for yourself or are you still working overtime?

Do you have trouble getting to sleep?

Are you aware of eating to alleviate stress or provide the illusion of pleasure?

Do you gulp down your food without tasting it?

If your answers to the majority of those questions indicate that you're living with chronic stress, you may want to consider changing your situation or yourself. You may be wondering how you can change yourself, but I assure you that you can, and in the chapters that follow I'll be providing you with the tools you need to do it.

Reassess Your Work Situation

If your work is confrontational or if it involves hurting people, it will tend to close you down emotionally. When that happens you may become detached, bored, and left with little pleasure. When you're starved for pleasure and emotional fulfillment you tend to overeat. If you're rushed, stressed, and constantly fatigued, you may make poor food choices and drink coffee just to get you through the day. The interaction between your eating habits and your choices at work can reveal how well or how poorly you and your work get along.

When you continue to work at a job that brings you few intellectual or emotional rewards your energy level will decrease and you'll have to push yourself harder and harder just to keep at it every day because you think you need to do that just in order to survive. If you keep asking yourself "how else will I survive?" you will begin to think less and less of yourself and you may begin to eat unhealthy foods or engage in addictive behaviors, all in a futile, counterproductive effort to make yourself feel better. If you're living in a decaying, unhappy, unhealthy work situation you need to think about changing either yourself or your work. Take a chance on trying one or the other.

You may be working too much or too hard because you're trying to live beyond your means. If you think that's what you're doing, you may need to reconsider your priorities. As the old saying goes, nothing else matters if you don't have your health.

Reassess Your Home Life

Are you relaxed at home? If not, is it because of your choices or the people around you? If you are abusing yourself at work, chances are you're doing the same at home. It's hard to turn off the tension and make that emotional switch. Is your home environment pleasant and peaceful?

Listen to Your Body

1   Are you carrying tension in your hands, your face, your jaw, or your neck? These are the places where tension usually resides. Noticing where you carry it will help you to consciously tell your body to let go of the tension.

2   Do your shoulders and head droop at the end of the day because you're worn out? If so, you're living with too much stress.

3   At the end of the day are you depressed or irritated? If so, what did you do with your day to leave you with those feelings?

Rebalance Your Priorities

If you can't change your work, you can change your approach to your work. You need to figure out how you can build pleasure into your work. But you also need to remember that you are not your job. You need to give yourself time to play, time to be creative, time to exercise, time to simply "be" without any obligations. Do you spend time looking at art, being in nature, interacting with animals or people? Do you use television or video games as substitutes for living? I guarantee you that there is no "reality" television and no simulated adventure to compare with really living your own life.

To help get to the root of your stress, take a good look at what you do with your time—on a daily, weekly, and yearly basis. Objectively examining your lifestyle can tell you a lot about yourself and is a tool you should use in conjunction with examining your thoughts and emotions. By doing that you'll have a better picture of how the two interact and will be better able to decide if you want or need to start doing anything differently. Don't spend the rest of your life stressed and simply surviving. You need to enjoy life and you can make that happen by making different choices. Change is at the heart of getting over whatever illness you might be experiencing; happiness is always your choice, no matter what your circumstances.

Make a plan; plan a change. Set a workout schedule. Set new mental, emotional, and physical goals. Start your day with a 5-minute meditation for confidence that everything will be okay, everything will get done. Be positive and give yourself a few minutes of mental and emotional clarity in the morning and a few minutes of relaxation and clarity at night.

Step Nine

START to Consider Your Thoughts and Your Emotions

Your thoughts and beliefs, your feelings and emotions lead you to be who you are and to do what you do. They are intimately tied to your overall health.

When you're floating along with great unexpected and unplanned success, you don't generally stop to consider why life is so good. Sometimes, however, life throws a monkey wrench in the works and you become ill or unhappy. Fortunately, when that happens, you can educate yourself to understand how you may have caused or contributed to the situation in which you find yourself. Most people don't really know how much their self-generated self-supportive or self-doubting thoughts influence what's happening in their lives.

Most Americans are not aware of the degree to which their thoughts and emotions directly impact their physical health. Your life history is largely dependent on how your mind works, and it just makes sense that the better you know yourself the better you'll be able to control and manage your life. Two people can live in the same surroundings and have quite different lives based on their internal, invisible "whys" of living. If you eat too much, why is that? If your life is unpleasant, why? If you are unmotivated or negative, why? These seem like pretty basic questions, but most of us never stop to consider them because we simply don't want to address the pain, self-criticism, or conflict that would entail.

Most people don't want to be made aware of their negative qualities, but it can actually be a relief to discover something about yourself that will help you make new choices and live a better, happier, healthier life. If you want to change, you need to evaluate yourself every so often.

Unreleased negative energy in the form of thoughts or beliefs and emotions are stored in the body and can eventually lead to disturbances on the cellular level. You can, however, be proactive by searching inside yourself and correcting those negative thoughts and beliefs that would otherwise manifest as or predispose you toward a physical illness.

Quantum physics has proved that mass (the physical body) and energy (thoughts and emotions) were not separate phenomena but could be converted to one another, and, furthermore, that the observer could actually affect the nature of what is observed. In terms of health and happiness, then, examining our thoughts and emotions and making an effort to change those that are not serving us well can and does affect what is happening in and to our body. Interestingly, the laws of quantum physics can be directly related to the ancient laws of karma, which hold that for every action there is an appropriate reaction, and that this holds true for mental and spiritual actions as well as for physical actions.

Most people want happiness, health, and a good home. You *can* have all that, and it really starts from the inside out, with your thoughts and emotional nature. You are what you think, and even old thoughts give rise to current emotions. You can have all good things once you discover what you may have been doing to sabotage yourself and why.

Contemplate Yourself

The best way to get to know yourself is simply to stop living moment to moment and take some time to consider why you do what you do. Do you have old childhood beliefs that may be limiting or harming you now? Do you have patterns of emotional reaction that may have helped you in the past but are not helping you now? You can continue to be damaged by old emotional injuries just as you can be damaged by a mental or emotional insult today. In the following chapter, "Using Contemplation, Meditation and Visualizations to Heal," I'll be providing you with the techniques that will help you to quiet the exterior noise so that you can focus inward, contemplate yourself, and rewrite the old subconscious tapes that may be limiting your happiness and success in the present.

Learn to Balance Your Head and Your Heart

There are head things and heart things, and in the United States we usually have too many head things going on—too many choices. We do too much thinking and not enough feeling. We need to find a balance between surviving from the head and living from the heart.

For most people, childhood offers the best examples of how to achieve that. Try to remember what it was like to be five or four or three years old and living with an undefended open exuberance for life. While you wouldn't want to live as an adult exactly the way you did as a child, there is much to be learned from seeing what you may unintentionally have left behind.

Do you go through your day fighting against feeling? We tend to resist being open and vulnerable to avoid being hurt, but that is a terrible way to go through life. Yes, we need to protect ourselves against an immediate danger, but once that danger has passed we need to open ourselves up and let our emotions fly. Think of yourself as a butterfly sailing with the wind instead of fighting it. If you have faith in the outcome, it can be a beautiful flight.

When you fight the wind or the world you start to have a sad, droopy face. You get lines and wrinkles from expressing the same negative emotions over and over again, and you do yourself other physical damage as well. To change your health, change your mind!

Step Ten

START to Consider a Fast

Once you've completed the previous 9 steps, you may want to consider fasting as a natural way to jumpstart regaining control of your health. Fasting gives your digestive system a time to rest, allows any immunologic processes triggered by food allergens time to resolve themselves, and—once your liver uses up it's glycogen stores—causes your body to begin burning fat for energy. In fact, the fat-burning produced by a fast works on exactly the same principles as a no-carb diet, only it does it through *natural* processes. In addition, the hormones released during fasting benefit both the mind and the body. The release of human growth hormone prepares your entire body to become leaner, and the endorphins produced by your brain will give you a kind of natural high with greater clarity. Many great thinkers of history, including Plato, Socrates, Confucius, Galen, Paracelsus, Christ, Moses, Muhammad, and Gandhi used fasting as a way to increase their self-knowledge and self-discipline, and to reveal higher motivations. Paracelsus, the great medieval physician, stated that fasting releases the physician within and brings out the natural healer. Consider also that all animals fast to heal. There is something about the many benefits of fasting that science is only beginning to discover.

I believe that the greatest benefit you will derive from a fast is the mental and emotional awareness it brings. By breaking the cycle of eating for pleasure or to release tension, a fast gives you the opportunity to consciously examine your day-to-day functioning and gain the insight into what drives and motivates you that will help you to change your life for the better.

Fasting is for people who want to directly take on reasons for illness and lessened health. With proper fasting you set a course that intensifies your mental, emotional and spiritual inquires into your psyche. It tends to bring your subconscious intelligence to consciousness, which can help you to set new goals and rebalance your life. It is a way to unblock and detox your mind and emotions at the same time you detoxify your body.

Although it isn't essential that you fast in order to contemplate and release the blocks that may exist in your mental and emotional life, without the power of fasting it might be more difficult to find and face the issues that have led you to ill health. Fasting is a powerful insight gatherer.

Why is Fasting the Last Step in the Change Process?

I believe that to get the most out of your fast you first need to prepare yourself physically, mentally, and emotionally. You need to cleanse your body of as many unnatural and incompatible foods and synthetic medications as you can and replace the nutrients you may have lost through eating poorly. You need to begin your self-education by looking into your lifestyle and thoughts. These preliminary nutritional and lifestyle changes will then allow you to get the most out of the mental and emotional benefits fasting can bring.

If you fast simply to lose weight, you will do that, but the change won't be long-lasting. If, on the other hand, you fast with the intention of seeking answers about your mental and emotional well-being, why you do what you do, your fast will press the reset button of your life and put you on the path to better living permanently.

In Chapter Eight I'll provide guidelines you need to undertake a safe and life-changing fast.

Ten Steps to Natural Health
Turn your Life Around

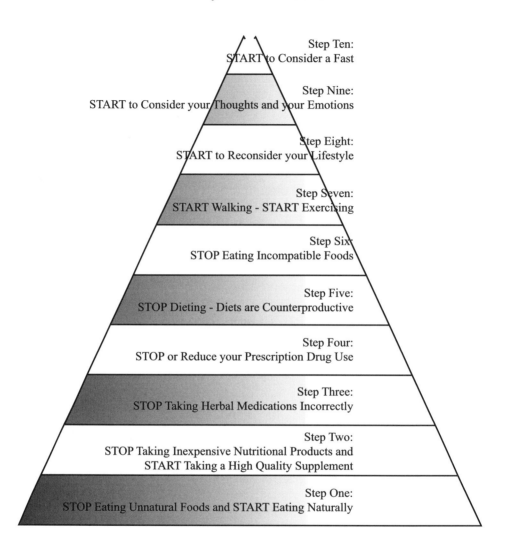

Step Ten:
START to Consider a Fast

Step Nine:
START to Consider your Thoughts and your Emotions

Step Eight:
START to Reconsider your Lifestyle

Step Seven:
START Walking - START Exercising

Step Six:
STOP Eating Incompatible Foods

Step Five:
STOP Dieting - Diets are Counterproductive

Step Four:
STOP or Reduce your Prescription Drug Use

Step Three:
STOP Taking Herbal Medications Incorrectly

Step Two:
STOP Taking Inexpensive Nutritional Products and
START Taking a High Quality Supplement

Step One:
STOP Eating Unnatural Foods and START Eating Naturally

Chapter Four

What Your Ancestors Can Teach You about Your Health

Although modern life brings us many conveniences and opens up possibilities our ancestors could never even have imagined, it has also taken us far from nature and the natural path to good health. To get you thinking about what that really means on the most basic level, let's take a look at what a day in the life of your prehistoric forebears might have been like.

The Morning Walk

Your ancestors would have awakened to morning sunshine and cool, clean air. They would have had to walk to the nearest source of water to drink. They wouldn't have been able to say, "I'm tired this morning. I think I'll skip my morning walk," because next to the need for air and protection from extreme heat and cold, your body needs water to maintain life. As they were walking, they were toning their muscles and stimulating the circulation of blood through their body. The morning air refreshed their lungs, brought movement to the diaphragm, and activated the colon. It also provided a peaceful time for being in nature and thinking about what the day might bring. A gentle morning walk preceded by a glass of water to replace what your body lost during the night of rest is the most natural way to start your day.

Most of us don't have access to the clean air our ancestors breathed every day, but we can still do our best to avoid inhaling toxic chemicals such as petroleum products, pesticides, herbicides, and insecticides that can damage brain cells and shorten lives. For city dwellers, in particular, I recommend using both a hepa filter and an ionic filter at home and at work.

The water your ancestors drank when they finally arrived at the stream contained no industrial pollutants. It was neither chlorinated nor fluorinated, and for the most part it had a high trace mineral content. It was oxygenated and free of electrical field charges. Whenever possible, drink mineralized water from a source that is free of environmental contaminants. Natural water has a vitality that stale bottled waters lack. You might need to filter your water to increase its purity.

Your ancestors would also have washed themselves in the stream, but they wouldn't have used harsh antibacterial soaps that alter the natural flora of the skin. Nor would they have used a stiff toothbrush that might introduce dental bacteria into the bloodstream and traumatize the gums. Unless you work in a job where you are exposed to dangerous bacteria, I don't recommend using anti-bacterial soap. And I suggest using a very soft toothbrush and stroking your gums in the direction of your teeth. You can also use a Waterpik to clean between your teeth.

Hunting and Gathering

The long drink of water your ancestors would have had at the stream would also have helped to curb their appetite. If you're in the habit of overeating, drinking a glass or two of water before meals will help to fill your stomach. It will also let you know if you've mistaken hunger for thirst.

Since they didn't have refrigerators to keep food fresh in their caves, they probably would have picked a light breakfast from a bush or a tree on the way home from the stream. Fruits, vegetables, and other plant sources of food were readily available, but they would have been eaten fresh and in season, and would have varied from month to month. They would not have been sprayed with pesticides or otherwise treated with chemicals, as most fruits and vegetables are today, and I, therefore, suggest that you wash your fruits and vegetables thoroughly or else discard the outer skins.

Your ancestors may have included grains in their morning meal, but they would have been different from the more modern grains we eat today, and they certainly wouldn't have been processed and served up in the form of a doughnut. Wheat entered the human diet relatively recently. More ancient grains—such as spelt, quinoa, and amaranth—are, therefore, more compatible with our digestion. Wheat, and particularly the gluten it contains, are incompatible with many people's bodies.

Other easily gathered foods would have been nuts (providing protein and fat) and eggs (for protein). Eggs are a whole protein, meaning that they contain all of the essential amino acids your body can't manufacture, so it is likely that eggs, in some form, entered the human diet very early.

To eat in a way that is most natural and compatible with your digestion, I would suggest a light vegetarian breakfast, which could be eggs, berries, or non-acidic fruit. If you're concerned with cholesterol, eat only the egg whites since all the cholesterol is contained in the yolks. And stay away from acidic (citrus) fruits (oranges, lemons, grapefruit) that can upset the acid/alkaline balance of your body and stress your kidneys. Citrus fruits have many healing qualities, but I recommend eating them in moderation. Coffee, sugar, and beer are also acidic. Cashews, almonds, garlic, broccoli, cabbage, peaches, and mangos are examples of alkaline foods. (See the Appendix for a list of common acid and alkaline foods.)

With all the effort involved in hunting, it's unlikely that your ancestors ate meat every day. Many days would have been totally vegetarian. For us modern humans, I recommend a sliding-scale diet of vegetarian/fish/fowl/lamb/pork/beef. Having said that, however, if you have a strong feeling about wanting to eat a particular food, you should have what you want. If you really want meat, eat it. But if you're trying to decide between vegetables and chicken, go for the vegetables. Every food that is produced naturally on this earth has some benefit for us.

Normally, fish, which is lean and full of essential fatty acids, would be the protein of choice. Today, however, I recommend that you avoid eating fish unless it is a short-lived small fish, you know it is from

Alaska, or you have a health report certifying that the fish is free of mercury and polychlorobiphenyls (synthetic herbicides and insecticides). Mercury has been linked to neurological damage in humans, and mercury contamination in fish is now almost universal.

Even if you choose an almost entirely vegetarian diet, however, you also need to make sure you're getting the proper nutritional balance. Unless you're very careful, vegetarian diets can be lacking in certain vitamins, amino acids, and essential fatty acids that you may need to take in the form of supplements. If you are deficient in any food nutrient, even one mineral, you may crave foods that contain what you're missing but are not otherwise healthy.

Where Did Your Ancestors Come From?

Although there are general rules about which foods to eat and which to avoid, you also need to remember that we all descend from different groups of ancestors and we each have a unique body chemistry. Foods that are native to wherever your parents and grandparents originate from are probably the ones you'll find most compatible with your body because they and your ancestors' DNA evolved together.

Among the foods known to be the most likely to cause allergic reactions are grains containing gluten (wheat, rye, barley, oats). These grains can be ideal for some and poison for others. To determine which category you fall into, you'll need to pay attention to your body and monitor your reactions to foods that contain them. Grain allergies can be the underlying cause of depression, migraines, epilepsy, and neurological disorders and have also been associated with diabetes, liver problems, thyroid disease, cancer, attention deficit disorder, and autism.

Another highly allergenic food is cow's milk and, consequently, dairy products that are derived from it. Cow's milk entered the human food chain relatively late in our development. We are better adapted to digesting other forms of dairy including goat and sheep milk products and yogurt, which is a bacterially altered form of cow dairy. In addition to yogurt, if you do use cow dairy, I suggest cottage cheese (also bacterially altered) and ghee, a purified form of butter.

Your Ancestors Didn't Have to Read Food Labels

Wherever your ancestors came from, their diet was comprised of foods created by Nature, not man. Since this is no longer the case, you need to know what to look for when you go into a food store. Generally speaking, anything that has a long, scientific name you can't pronounce is something you should avoid. Beyond that, stay away from artificial flavors or flavor enhancers (such as msg), artificial sweeteners, or coloring agents.

Among ingredients that may sound natural but that should be avoided are high fructose corn syrup, hydrogenated oils, and long chain oils including cottonseed and canola oils.

Although "fructose" sounds healthy, high fructose corn syrup is actually a man-made product derived from corn and processed to increase the amount of fructose in the syrup. Although the processing is complicated, the end product is actually cheaper than sugar and is, therefore, used by manufacturers in everything from sodas to jams to snack foods. Many researchers have found an association between our increased consumption of high fructose corn syrup and the increase in obesity and type 2 diabetes in America.

Similarly, cottonseed oil, palm kernel oil, and canola oil are oils not normally found in the food chain. Because they increase shelf life and are less expensive than other, healthier types of oil, they are now in many, many products including most chips and cereals.

The oils I recommend using are cold-pressed sunflower and olive oil or coconut oil for cooking. You may also want to try avocado oil, flax oil, sesame oil, or walnut oil. I recommend staying away from peanut oil because peanuts are so highly allergenic to so many people. Try not to heat oils beyond 360 degrees because they become carcinogenic at high temperatures and store them in a dark place or wrapped in aluminum foil to avoid their turning rancid.

The Natural Cycle of Sleep

Despite its dangers, your ancestors' life was a lot simpler than yours is today. They would have had a last drink of water and been back in their shelter before dark. They wouldn't have had a glass or two of water and a snack before going to sleep. As a result, they probably enjoyed better digestion, a good night's sleep, and better elimination. To enjoy the same degree of natural bodily cycles, you'd probably benefit from not eating or drinking after 8 pm.

The amount of physical activity they engaged in would have helped to increase circulation and encouraged detoxification while also releasing the endorphins that help us to relax and sleep well. Since we are no longer forced to walk or run to find water and catch our food on the hoof, we need to get moving in other ways. If you don't naturally enjoy or engage in a sport or physical activity, make one up. Walk up and down the halls, dance around your office, swim, ride a bike, take ballroom dancing classes. Just find some way to fit physical activity into your lifestyle.

But it's not only exercise that helped your ancestors to sleep well. They also had less stress in their lives. Certainly there were stressful moments—such as being chased by a wild animal—but once the danger was gone, so was the stress. Modern stress, on the other hand, is much more pervasive and insidious. We live so much in our heads that we internalize our emotions instead of expressing and releasing them in the moment. These bottled-up feelings then fester within us until they manifest as physical ailments and/or prevent us from enjoying peaceful, restorative sleep.

According to some estimates, between 50 percent and 70 percent of Americans do not sleep well. In addition to poor diet and lack of exercise, one of the primary causes of this epidemic of sleep-deprivation is mental and emotional overload. Taking sleep medications will not get to the root of the problem and may, in fact, cause additional problems including fuzzy thinking and drug dependency.

In Chapter Six you will find exercises for dumping the excess thoughts and emotions that may be preventing you from sleep. You will also find that the healthier you become both physically and emotionally, the less sleep you'll need. So, if you find that you are sleeping a lot or are tired all the time, you are probably trying to heal something you may not even be aware of harboring.

Try to Live More Naturally

Your ancestors lived naturally from necessity. For us, living more naturally must be a conscious choice. We can choose to eat more natural foods, to avoid as many medications as possible, and to pay attention to our bodies, our thoughts, and our emotions.

We can also choose to change habits that are not serving us well. Take a walk instead of plopping down in front of the television every night. Turn a deaf ear to the constant barrage of advertising that encourages us to buy things we don't need. Consider making changes in our work or home situation that may be causing too much stress.

We can't go back to living in caves, but we can take a cue from our ancestors and try to live more as they did, which will be more compatible with the way our bodies have evolved.

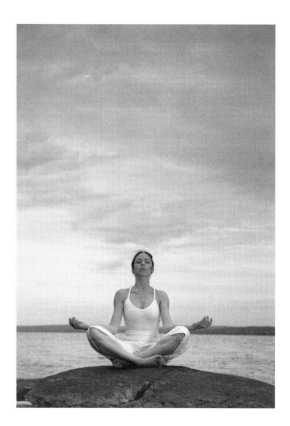

Plant the Seeds of Good Health

in your Mind.

Chapter Five

Using Contemplation, Meditation, and Visualizations to Heal

The link between your body and your mind is active every day, even though you may not be aware of how your thoughts and emotions, both past and present, are affecting your physical health.

Suppressed thoughts and feelings manifest as physical symptoms, which means that if you're feeling bad you need to uncover and correct the negative thoughts and emotions that exist below the level of consciousness. If your life is going great you might not need to spend time evaluating how it got that way. But if the past has limited your present and future, you need to look into past thoughts, ideas, and ways of living that may be affecting you today. Having done that, you'll be able to combine the best of the old with the best of what you learned to create a better future.

Connecting with Your Inner Wisdom

When you're seeking the cause of a physical ailment, its original cause might be a belief you hold about something or yourself, it might be an emotional imprint you implanted in your body and subconscious, or it might be a habitual way of acting or reacting. Once you understand the original cause, you will have the awareness that gives you the ability to make new choices.

I should emphasize here that in considering your beliefs and drives, there should be no blame or guilt attached to your seeking. You are looking only for causality. You may need to look for why you tend to blame others or why you feel guilty or afraid, but you're doing that only to discover where those traits came from, not in order to judge. When you are able to do that, you will have connected with your inner wisdom. Three of the most effective means of doing this are contemplation, meditation, and visualization.

Contemplation is not just for old people sitting on park benches. Meditation is not just for balding wise men in robes sitting on top of mountains. Visualization is not voodoo. Anyone can contemplate, meditate, and visualize a better future. Often, you need to start by contemplating your past. You don't need any special equipment. All you need is yourself, some solitude and some time. Nutritional purity will help you.

Will contemplation, meditation, and visualization earn you money or get you dates? Well, not immediately. But the changes and growth that come from truly getting to know yourself connection with your inner wisdom will bring you more accomplishment and fulfillment than you can imagine. Ultimately, what you gain in knowing and balancing yourself can lead you away from illness to healthy, joyful living.

Contemplation

Contemplation is considering a question or situation and letting insightful thoughts come to mind. Contemplating something involves thinking, but it is more than thinking *about* something. It is pondering a particular question and listening for answers. It is a way of gazing intently with your inner vision and listening with your inner ear. It involves silently asking "why?"

When you contemplate yourself you are using a part of your mind to examine your mind. It requires that you use your intellect but also calls upon your greater intelligence—your thoughts moving in harmony with your feelings, your memory, and your intuition. You can use this greater intelligence to identify and explain what does or doesn't motivate you, why it is that you do what you do. The more you use the technique and make changes based on your discoveries about yourself, the more you will begin to notice your emotional patterns and understand how they were originally imprinted on your psyche.

Taking charge of your thoughts in this way brings with it great responsibility. It is taking charge of your own destiny, and that's a responsibility many people really don't want. It seems safer somehow just to drift across the sea of life without ever putting your hand on the rudder. Going with the flow can seem very peaceful until an ill wind blows your ship toward the rocks. When that happens, however, you may want to take charge and change course before you wind up shipwrecked.

How to Contemplate

First, find a time when you will not be disturbed and a place where you can create peace and clarity. It could be as close as your own bedroom or someplace out in the country. Generally, it's also a good idea to decide in advance what specific issue you're going to contemplate. In the beginning you will likely have many choices.

As you begin, many other thoughts or subjects will come to mind. Dismiss them and stay focused. It's important that you delve deeply into your issues one at a time and follow one subject to its source before moving on. With each answer that comes up, keep asking "why" until you feel comfortable that you have the final answer. If you open up too many issues at once without completely resolving any of them, you'll just become even more confused.

Let's say you begin with the question, "Why am I overweight?" Your first answers might be, "I'm so stressed out," "I never have any fun," or "My spouse/partner doesn't love me anymore." Deeper questions and answers come from contemplating the first ones. So, if one of your answers was "I'm so stressed out," your next question might be, "Why am I so stressed out?" Contemplate that and, when you have an answer, go on to the next "why."

You might learn that you're stressed because you're so hypercritical and never satisfied with the work you do. Give yourself a moment to feel the truth of that and then ask again, "Why?" You might discover that you've been hypercritical of yourself ever since you were sixteen years old. "Why?" Maybe at that age your first boyfriend dumped you or your parents were pressuring you to get high grades. Keep going and contemplate any negative issues that arise until you can't trace the origin back any further.

As you contemplate a past negativity or rejection you may discover that your sense of self-worth was lowered or eroded at that time. You may have begun to protect yourself from some imagined further hurt by keeping people at arm's length and not making yourself vulnerable to intimacy.

At this point you may be wondering why on earth you would want to begin exploring all these dark caves of your mind to discover what's hidden inside. That's perfectly normal, but what you need to remember is that if you want to change for the better, you'll have to take at least a few steps outside your comfort zone. There's no right or wrong way to do that. You can laugh or cry. Give yourself breaks when you need them.

If you've been holding onto your old, negative thoughts and beliefs, they will continue to fill you with negative energy that may manifest as pain or nausea when it is released. Don't fight it or try to minimize it; let the feelings out completely. Release them from your body and give yourself permission to heal and feel good.

The final step of your contemplation will be to use positive self-talk and affirmations to erase and record over the old, faulty tape or belief that's been stuck inside you. You don't actually have to talk out loud, but you do need to engage in a focused and determined dialogue with yourself.

When you've uncovered the event or belief from the past that is causing you to act or react the way you do in the present, ask yourself if you would like to change it. For example, if you've discovered that you always snack when you read because your father used to pressure you to read when you were a child and the pleasure of the snacking helped you to deal with the pressure of his insisting that you read, you need to decide if you can accept reading without snacking and if you can deal with pressure without eating. Tell yourself that eating to deal with pressure is making you sick, overweight, and unhappy. Keep reminding yourself of this until the need for change is deeply implanted in your mind. Then switch to the positive and reinforce nurturing habits. Always conclude with the positive.

Once you've done that, have a dialogue between your present self and your child self. Speak with compassion. Remember that your reaction to the situation (eating to relieve the pressure of reading) may have served a purpose in the past but that you now want to change it. Acknowledge that your father wanted you to succeed, which was a good thing, and how good it felt to feel his love. Feel grateful that he encouraged you to read, but, at the same time, assert your present choice to take responsibility for your reading and respond to it in a healthier manner. No one is pressuring you and you don't need food. Keep repeating the positive words until you are comfortable with them. Consciously raise your level of self-worth, and tell yourself that you desire and deserve to be happy. Life has pressures and stresses, but you can handle them and you will be alright! Change the frequency of your energy from negative to positive. Keep repeating the words, "Everything will be alright," and it will be.

Continue to revisit and repeat your self-talk conversation until you have fully accepted the changes you're making. Remember that it took many years for you to become who you are, so it can take a little time to reverse or over-write old destructive thoughts and habits. Be patient. Speak to yourself sincerely, logically, and with kindness. Your mind can accept logic and kindness just as well as it accepts illogic and pain.

You will discover that contemplating one issue often yields insights into other issues. You might, for example find that several other behaviors lead back to your feeling a lack of self-worth. Maybe realizing that you eat to reward yourself will help you to realize that you avoid inviting certain people to dinner because you don't feel you deserve their company or because you're protecting yourself from their potential criticism. Every behavior has a root cause, and the more of them you can uncover the more completely you'll be able to change your old subconscious patterns. Tracking down and uncovering the origins of your feelings and thoughts is key to changing the patterns of your life. It is by consciously, willfully taking responsibility that you take true control of your body and your mind.

Everyone's life involves some difficulty and pain. We all face challenges and even disasters. But not everyone needs to respond to negative events by becoming depressed, angry, or overweight. With a little more self-awareness you can, with time, learn to respond differently when life throws you a curve. By doing that you will feel more joy and have more control, which means more freedom, in your life. It is truly an issue of mind over matter. But, unlike counting calories or going on a diet, this kind of control will create permanent change.

Specific Issues You Might Want to Contemplate

Contemplate why you eat, especially if it is excessive. If, like so many people, you are overweight you might want to look into what triggers your eating. Do you eat for pleasure or to alleviate anxiety? Are you bored or eating to be social? If so you might want to ask yourself what other activities you might engage in that would alleviate your boredom and increase your sociability without harming your body. Some people eat because they fear intimacy and want to hide. Some people just want to push down their feelings. Whatever negative emotion is triggering your eating, you need to uncover it so that you can release it.

If you've failed at something you tried, you might want to contemplate what benefit you derive from failing. Do you get pity or compassion from others or yourself. Do you have such a need for sympathy and kindness that you simply can't risk success? Does failing give you permission to eat more? Do you believe that your success will make others feel worse? Get a pad and pencil and, on one side of the page, list all the things you've been getting from failure. Then, on the other side of the page, list all the things you could be getting if you allowed yourself to succeed.

Contemplate why you get angry. What pushes your buttons? What threats to your dreams and desires cause you to get angry? What happens when you get angry? If you are frequently angry, take a look at the reasons and ask yourself whether your anger improved the situation or damaged your relationships. Getting to the core of your anger will show you how it works and, therefore, how to control it. First, however, you must figure out how to release and let go of it so that it doesn't continue to build up and block your positive energy. The best ways to do this are to:

1   Understand that it is a purely emotional reaction and not proof that you are right.

2   Notice other people's perspective and the situations that trigger your anger.

3   Redirect your feelings of anger into less hurtful and more useful channels.

Contemplate how you deal with accepting and expressing intimacy. Consider how much true intimacy you have in your life. How deeply do you share your thoughts and feelings with another person. When you withhold or cannot accept intimacy, you may turn to eating as a safe way to satisfy or stuff down your emotions. You may be choosing to eat heavy, fatty foods that require a lot of energy for digestion—leaving that much less energy for you to deal with your thoughts and emotions. If you're aware of this behavior in yourself, look within for the ability to become more open and express your feelings to others. Allowing yourself the intimacy of even a simple conversation can bring you so much contentment that you may immediately have less need or desire to eat. Satisfying your heart is a requirement for healthy living.

Contemplate your parents. Because our parents are the first people we observed, they provided our primary example of how to live. We naturally react and behave like our parents more than we know. Just as most people retain the religious and political beliefs that were handed down to them, so do we customarily accept our inherited ways of thinking and reacting. If you're not happy with the choices you've made for yourself, you may want to consider that they probably weren't choices at all—or, at least not conscious choices. Contemplate the good in your parents and gratefully affirm those qualities that are in you. Realistically assess those qualities in your parents that were ineffective and that you see in yourself and choose to let them go.

Contemplate your likes and dislikes. What gives you pleasure? What causes you pain? Write them down and see if you can distill what you've written into a few basic, core drives. Doing that will help you to discover what motivates you, which will, in turn, help you to make better choices for yourself. Knowing, for example, that you don't like being alone may lead you to choose a more satisfying vocation or avocation in the future. Looking more deeply, you may find that you're still missing your mother, who left when you were ten years old. This might explain why you're attracted to emotional, demonstrative people who may be providing the nurturing you didn't get as a child. You don't have to be that limited!

Contemplate how truthfully you express yourself to others. Do you represent yourself as you truly are or do you show a mask to the world? Do you know how to ask for what you truly need? Do you even know what you need? Do you need to own things because you don't express yourself in a way that would bring you other things—companionship, joy, peace—that you really need more?

Contemplate the role competition plays in your life. Very often the need to compete results from and/or reinforces low self-esteem. If you are competitive, consider why you feel that need. Maybe the one you're really competing with is yourself. Consider how competition may have negatively affected your relationships when other people have "lost" to you. The competitive drive can be harmful both to you and to others.

Contemplate your dreams. You'll be amazed how easily you can draw conclusions from the situations and people in your dreams. Keep a pad and pencil by your bed and write them down as soon as you awaken so that you'll be able to contemplate them at leisure. Be aware that everyone in your dream may represent some aspect of you. You may also want to consult a dream book to help you figure out the meaning of a particular dream. If a situation in your dream is extremely emotional, it generally means that you're harboring those emotions on an unconscious level in your life and that you need to become aware of them so that you can release them.

Meditation

Meditation is both like and unlike contemplation. Whereas in contemplation you are purposefully thinking about a specific issue or situation in order to get answers from and about yourself, in meditation your goal is to stop your mind from thinking by focusing on a particular word, image, phrase, or feeling. You are quieting the conscious part of your mind in order to give your subconscious mind more freedom to emerge.

In meditation you transcend your normal conscious awareness in order to achieve a higher level of consciousness. It's one thing to use your conscious, thinking mind to get you through everyday life, but sometimes you can overuse it, especially when you can't stop or control your thoughts. Runaway, discursive thinking, especially when you're under pressure, can lead you to make poor choices and to act unkindly. By slowing or actually stopping those thoughts, you can become more connected to your emotions. By quieting your mind you open your heart. When an unsettled mind is controlling you, your direction is unclear; when you still the mind, you gain self-control and know which way to go.

Learning to meditate is probably more important today than at any time in human history. With so many technological advances, we are daily presented with endless possibilities and our minds are working so continuously and so fast that our hearts sometimes get left behind. We lack balance and, as a result, we can become overwhelmed, confused, depleted, and depressed. We have so many choices that we wind up doing nothing. We need to free ourselves from the chaos and let our thoughts reconnect with our hearts.

How to Meditate

If you've already used contemplation to become more familiar with your subconscious beliefs and emotions, you've been developing the patience and diligence you will need for meditation. In addition to those qualities you will also need focused attention and openness to insight.

As with contemplation you need to find a quiet time and place where you will not be disturbed. You can meditate in any position, even lying down, but I suggest, at least the beginning, that you remain sitting up so that you don't inadvertently fall asleep. Sleeping may feel good, but it will leave you short of the mark.

A good way to start is to discipline your mind by giving it just one task or image to focus on. This is called single point meditation. Your mind, as you probably found out during your contemplations, has a tendency to wander. When you learn to still your mind, you open yourself up to a deeper level of intelligence.

A single point meditation can be as simple as focusing on a particular color. Sit in a comfortable position and place a color—blue, for example—before your mind's eye. Focus on seeing the color blue and nothing else. Your mind will undoubtedly wander. When that happens, acknowledge the thought, let it be okay, and dismiss it. You may become uncomfortable and want to move. Keep returning your focus to blue. It may take some time to train your mind to do this, but when you can maintain the color in front of you until you stop thinking about time, you will have achieved a meditative state. You may derive no great meaning from this at first, but you will have begun to train your mind to be still and brought order to the chaos most of us live with everyday.

If you prefer to do an aural meditation, you can repeat a single word or sound, such as om, or love, or peace, either aloud or in your mind until you have lost track of time but still remain conscious.

You may, in fact, have experienced something like this in your everyday life, when, for example, you were in your car and driving for perhaps hours at a time, stopping, turning, accelerating without consciously thinking about what you were doing or about the passage of time. Distance runners can also experience this meditative state, often referred to as being "in the zone."

It may take a while for you to develop the ability to voluntarily slow and stop your thoughts. Don't be discouraged. There may be long periods of time when you experience no significant breakthrough, and then, suddenly, it comes. Just your sincere effort and faith in the outcome will elevate your nature and open your heart.

Advanced Meditations

As you become more comfortable with and adept at the practice you can try more complex forms of meditation. Only the subject of your focus will change; the process remains the same.

You might, for example, choose to meditate on the meaning of the world. Start thinking about the world; hold a feeling or image of the world in your mind until you have lost track of time. As intelligent or scientifically trained as you may believe yourself to be, a successful meditation will show you how much more knowledge lies within you. The more you meditate, the more you will allow those hidden and invisible truths to come through.

The Seeing and Knowing Meditation: This is an exercise in which you choose an object, such as a clear vase or a clay pot, to look at. Stare at the object and see it's shape and color. If you wish, you can feel the texture with your fingers. Now expand your way of "seeing" the object. See it in three dimensions; notice its location in the world. Imagine seeing deeper into its texture so that you feel the individual materials of which it is made. Start to incorporate the "feel" of the object into your own body so that you feel as it does. This type of meditation can bring your mind into greater alignment with the world around you, making you more observant and patient.

Emotional Meditation: You can introduce emotion into your meditations. For example, after doing one of the exercises dealing with joy in Chapter Six, meditate about joy or the feeling of joy. Feel the energy and sensation of joy as you meditate. Willfully increase and spread the joy throughout your body and consciousness. Afterward, pay attention to yourself. You may notice some interesting improvements in your body. Experiencing joy is important for your overall health and success.

Conceptualization Expansion: Pick an idea or concept to meditate on. You might, for example, pick the concept of space. To consider space, stand in a room with mirrors on either side. Notice how you can look in one mirror and see infinite mirror images of yourself. Consider what is real. Consider physical space and outer space. In your imagination you can travel to other planets, stars, and galaxies. You can continue doubling outer space into infinity. Now shift your focus to considering a molecule and then an atom. Continue to halve each micro-distance. There is no end to how small you can make something.

This type of meditation can make you aware of the illusion of physical space. Spirit goes on forever, and that is what you really are. Not an image in a mirror. Probing this kind of concept will expand the possibilities of your mind.

Meditate on Nothing: Stay conscious and allow your mind to stop producing thoughts. The best way to do this is probably to focus your awareness on listening to everything around you. The single point is both nothing and everything at once. If you start to think of any one specific thing, keep bringing yourself back to nothingness.

Visualizations

Visualization is a way to broadcast your goals to enhance your chances of achieving them. You can, for example, visualize your future self joyful and free of any ailment. You can use this technique for anything you want to achieve, but I would caution against visualizing harmful acts when you see yourself in the future. Although your visualization may seem rather abstract at first, you will notice that it has a powerful, tangible effect on your mind. Do a visualization as often as you can. Many of the emotional exercises in the following chapter use visualization as part of the process, and you may find that your visualizing the future will be enhanced if you do it following one of these exercises. The visualization can last anywhere from one to five minutes.

Seated comfortably or lying down, close your eyes and imagine yourself in the future doing exactly what you would like to be doing. See yourself at peace with everything around you, in an environment entirely of your choosing, healthy and free of pain. See yourself open-minded and giving love freely and receiving it from others. See yourself happy.

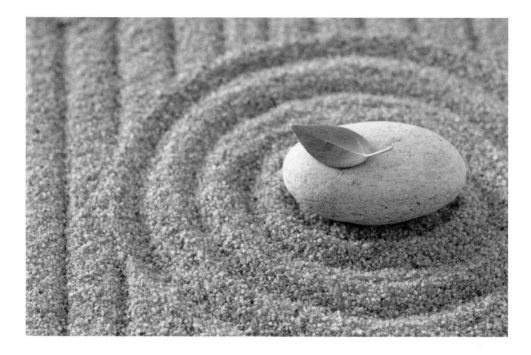

Loving

and

Healing

Chapter Six

Healing Emotional Exercises

Love, faith, and hope are real and essential for the health of your body, mind, and spirit. Therefore, integrating and balancing your thoughts and feelings will contribute to your health, and the *types* of thoughts and emotional energies that predominate will eventually manifest in your physical body. The exercises in this chapter will help you to release the unnecessary negative thoughts and feelings you may be holding onto from your past so that you can experience the peace and well-being that help you to heal. While being positively focused is important 90 percent of the time, it can become necessary to intentionally release negativity when it blocks your natural flow of well-being.

In addition, exercises that consciously expand your awareness and focus on other people and things will help you to become a more selfless person who is more aware of the "non-you" than the you. Too much criticism or too much time spent on healing yourself can lead to selfishness or self-absorption, so I offer exercises that will create other-awareness and release compassion, which are necessary for true humanity and evolution of the spirit.

Although the exercises that follow may have simple-sounding names they involve profoundly important inner principles that deal with rebalancing your spirit—something that is rarely considered by science with relation to health. They go beyond merely making you aware of a problem by allowing you actually to go inside yourself and manipulate your principles.

The Wake Up Exercise

This exercise takes less than 20 seconds. It's designed to do in the morning, before you get out of bed, as a way to reintegrate your body with your sense of touch, but you can do it anytime you feel the need to reconnect with your body and your sense of yourself. Normal blood flow moves from inside to out, and this exercise actually re-circulates the stagnant blood that collects in your extremities while you sleep.

From a supine position, reach down and put your hands around one of your feet. Push down and gently compress your skin as you slowly pull your hands up toward your waist. By wrapping your hands around your leg and thigh as you come up, you are literally pushing the blood in your superficial veins ahead as you go. Repeat the process with the opposite leg. Then slide one hand up the opposite arm, pressing the skin as you move upward and over your shoulder. Do the same with the other hand and arm. Next, press your hands against your waist, moving them upward across your back, then up your sides and abdomen, reaching forward toward your heart. Finally, pressing more lightly, go over your neck, your face, and up toward the top of your head. Even though the blood from your head moves down toward your heart, moving your hands upward across your facial muscles and scalp sets your expression in a smiling, "happy" position and similarly realigns your physical sense of well-being.

Don't leave out any part of your body. All of you needs to feel connected and in balance.

The Thought-Extinguishing Exercise

Modern society presents us with so many difficult choices to make and obligations to keep, and we have so much time to think that sometimes our minds feel literally overloaded. Interestingly enough, most of what's going on in our mind and causing us stress is self-generated. While you may think that whatever is causing your mind to work overtime is coming at you from the outside world, the majority of it comes from your on-going effort to protect yourself from something that *might* happen, although about 90 percent of the things we spend our time worrying about will never come to pass. This kind of self-generated stress can lead to chronic fatigue, delusional thinking, and/or inappropriate behavior. This is a problem you can't actually see or touch but it is one of the most health-damaging aspects of modern society.

Mental overload may, in fact, be one of the primary reasons we become overweight and out of shape. That's why it's so important to empty your thoughts at bedtime. If you have too much on your mental plate, you'll sleep poorly and end up spending most of your dream-time just eliminating your leftover thoughts and worries. That can make for some very strange dreams, such as having a conversation with your boss at a movie theater or trying to make your sales quota while dining at a restaurant. You can do this exercise during the day if you feel yourself going into mental overload, but for the most part it's designed to do at bedtime to help you enjoy better health and a good night's sleep.

Start by making yourself comfortable, either lying down or sitting. Take a few deep breaths and let your muscles relax. Imagine a warm and comforting campfire in front of you and stare into the flames. Place whatever thoughts come to you into the fire. You can imagine them as having shape and form if you wish. One by one, look at each thought and then see it burn away in the fire, going up in smoke. This will take anywhere from five to twenty minutes, depending on how many thoughts come into your mind.

If imagining the fire is a problem for you, you might feel more comfortable picturing yourself standing by a river and letting your thoughts wash downstream. Or, you could stand on a mountain top and let your thoughts be blown away with the wind. Whatever image allows you to release your thoughts so that you feel relaxed and peaceful is fine.

If any particular thought offers resistance and keeps coming back to you, tell yourself that you don't have to deal with it right then; you can be reminded of it in the morning. Take a deep breath and let it out, mentally affirming that all situations work themselves out eventually. This might help you to let go of that difficult thought. In the world of thought, what makes some imagined outcome a problem is believing that it will happen. Why do that? Let it be. Your mind must empty at night in order to heal.

The Breath and Pulse Countdown Exercise

This exercise, like the previous one, will reduce your level of stress. In addition, it will help your body develop the ability to respond more easily to your thoughts and feelings. You will be increasing your body-awareness while putting yourself into a deep, restful state, which will also prepare you for whatever kind of biofeedback you may ever need to do. The exercise takes ten to twenty minutes.

Once again, assume a comfortable position. If it's chilly, put on a sweater or wrap a blanket around your shoulders. Begin to focus on your breathing, preferably breathing through your nose. Then, begin to concentrate less directly on your breathing but sense your chest moving up and down. The natural way to breathe is from very deep in the abdomen, so as you relax, your breathing will shift from your chest to deeper abdominal breathing. Just let it be easy and relaxed.

As you relax, gradually allow yourself to breathe more slowly. Start to let a little more time pass after you exhale and before you inhale again. It doesn't matter if the size of your breaths is irregular. You may begin to feel sleepy, but don't let yourself fall asleep before you've completed the exercise.

Remaining relaxed and focused, remain aware of the rate of your breathing and let it slow down. After two to five minutes, let your breathing slow down again and begin to concentrate on your heartbeat. Get a sense of your heart's rate of contraction, but don't actually count your heartbeats because doing that will interfere with your relaxation.

Just notice each beat and generally be aware of the pace. Once you get a steady feeling, think about letting your heart slow down; just form the idea without any expectation of time frame. You will feel yourself breathing more deeply and your heart slowing down even more. Slowly and comfortably instruct your heart to go even slower as you lead it into more and more relaxed rhythms. The tension will release from your body as you do this. Maintain this slow steady state for as long as you like, and, when you're finished, you can, if you want, fall asleep.

The Age Count-Back Exercise

This age-related memory exercise enhances the self-discoveries you've made through your contemplations and meditations. It will help you to determine when you began to feel certain ways, when you made a significant change in the way you think, what happened to you at an earlier age that affected your life significantly. The exercise will take from fifteen to forty-five minutes and can also be done in reverse, counting forward from some specific younger age.

Certain of your opinions about your own worth, your abilities, intelligence, and courage may have been created at various times in your life. It's therefore useful, when you do this exercise, to have in mind some particular belief or feeling whose origin you want to discover. You can do it over and over again for as many beliefs as you would like to uncover and change.

For example, you might be aware that you're a negative and

pessimistic person, and would like to change those feelings because they're driving people away and, moreover, your pessimism is becoming a self-fulfilling prophesy, leading you to fail in your job or relationships. You remember that you weren't always so negative, and you want to find out what caused you to change your outlook. Once you've done that, you'll be able to change it. Whatever your mind created, your mind has the ability to change.

To begin, find a comfortable position, preferably lying down. Close your eyes and recall your life as of this month. Describe aloud or to yourself how you feel and what's going on. Then do the same for the previous year. For example, your self dialogue might be, "It's 2005 and I'm working at a job I don't like. I'm seeing Cathy (or Mike) and it's going alright although I know our relationship suffers because I'm so negative."

Keep going back, year by year, as far as you need to. As you continue to do this, eventually you'll come to a time—probably during your youth or school days—when you didn't act or feel the way you are now. At that point, hone in on the time of year, the month, even the day if you can, and start to recall specific events. The triggering event may have been obviously traumatic, such as the death of a loved one, or it may be something that is apparently innocuous and unimportant. However big or small, it doesn't matter. What matters is how it affected you.

You will usually uncover events, people, and circumstances that you know are linked to your current belief or behavior. When you get to the specifics, however, you will come to understand that in that moment you misinterpreted something that led to the way you are now. No matter how untrue it may be, if you hold a negative belief about yourself you will manifest it in your life.

To change these beliefs, once you've gotten to the source and understood how, at the time, you could have concluded whatever it is about yourself, you can begin to tell yourself that you made a mistake, that your feelings have changed, and that you want to be different. You want and deserve to be happy; you want to notice and validate positive qualities in others. And because you want to be happy, you will project positive images of your future. You will know that if something doesn't work out, you'll still be okay. Not only do you see the world with your eyes, you also project onto it with your inner vision thoughts and beliefs that color not only how you see what's going on around you but also how others see you. Self-talk is extremely important once you've gotten to the source of your old beliefs so that you can affirm the new belief to your deepest core.

To reinforce your new, positive feelings and perspectives, you might want to find a tangible reminder you can look at throughout the day. For example, you could buy a butterfly key chain because the butterfly is a symbol of joy and freedom. Or maybe you'd prefer a dragonfly, which symbolizes change. Eventually you'll find that you no longer need reminders or gadgets to reinforce your new outlook on yourself and your life.

The Four-Year-Old Exercise

Following the Age-Countdown Exercise you might want to do this one to recapture the natural energy, openness, and joy you had as a four-year-old. It can take from five to thirty minutes.

Lie down, focus, and concentrate. Remember or imagine your life and feelings at the open and jubilant age four. Think of a place you would have been, things you would have done—playing, having fun, looking at the world with a sense of wonderment.

Now, get up and move around. Play-act being a child again. Skip, hop, sing. You will be emotionally rejuvenated.

When you're done, assess your feelings and emotions and compare them to your current state of being. What keeps you from your youthful joy and freedom of expression? Are your adult defenses and beliefs really serving you and making you happy? Are you afraid of what others think of you? Hmm. Reconnect with the equally important and vitally passionate emotions of your youth.

The Anger-Releasing Exercise

Although some researchers would say that anger-releasing methods such as punching a pillow only lead to the creation of more anger, I believe that this is not necessarily true. So many people have built-up anger that once they tap into it and release it, it feels good to release even more. While I certainly don't recommend hitting people or surrounding yourself with anger, I do believe in the absolute value of releasing this damaging emotional energy. The exercise can take anywhere from five minutes to one hour. After completing the exercise, it would be a good idea to augment its benefits by doing the Thought Extinguishing Exercise, and/or engaging in some positive self-talk, and repeating affirmations of joy.

It would also be a good idea to take a close look at why you've built up all this anger. You don't want to wind up punching the pillow so routinely that you have no place left to put your head down. And expressing your anger at a person or a problem may be only a temporary solution; you might really need to change the situation or change whatever it is in you that's causing you to allow it to happen.

Our minds tend to imagine and then manifest situations that allow us to expend our built-up anger, so that the angrier we are, the more negative we become, and the more bad outcomes, frustration, and missed opportunities we bring into our lives. That said, at some time every one of us is going to find him- or herself at the bottom of the pecking order, being dumped on or picked on by everyone in our life. When that happens to you, you effectively have no one on whom to transmit your own accumulated anger. Or maybe you just don't believe that there should be a pecking order; you don't believe in passing on your own negativity. That's a very noble attitude, and it would be great if you weren't accepting and storing all the negative energy being dumped on you and into your body like a toxic substance.

This exercise is also extremely useful for getting rid of anger left over from the past. If, for example, someone hurt you or wronged you and that person is no longer around, you can still act out your hostility privately and productively.

Our society generally disapproves of anger, causing us to "stuff down" our emotions instead of expressing them. If you're in that position, it wouldn't be unusual for you to try to counter all that negativity with the "safe" pleasure of overeating or engaging in other so-called safe but actually harmful activities.

What actually would be safer, and far more productive would be to practice the Anger Releasing Exercise followed by a pleasure- or joy-enhancing exercise such as the "4 year old exercise" or the "self-loving exercise" to bring more positive energy into your life.

Before we begin, a word of caution: Don't do this exercise in a place or at a time when your yelling is going to be disturbing to anyone else.

Find someplace private and do one or more of the following things: Imagine the person you're angry at in the room with you. Yell at him or her loudly and with your full diaphragm. Shake your fists. Kick and shout. I also recommend punching a pillow. Make sure it's big and sturdy enough to take a good punch and made of a material that won't hurt your hands. Punch it, kick it, step on it, while telling it every angry thing you need to get out. You might not even be angry at a specific person. Maybe you're just angry with life or the world. Shake your fists and generally allow yourself to do whatever it is that will release your anger and make you feel like you've dumped your emotional load.

Afterwards you'll feel very relaxed. I actually once had a client who worked at an S & M club where she hit other people for their peculiar pleasure. I'm not saying that I approve either of hitting people or of her particular career path, but I do know that this woman was one of the calmest, most relaxed people I've ever met. Because of her work, she regularly released more negative energy than normal life would have allowed.

The Giant Will-Stomping Exercise

This exercise will help you to assert your will in a resistant world. It is in part derived from Dr. Lee Lipsenthal, MD. Use it when you make a plan but find it difficult to implement or when you need to affirm your perspective in a difficult situation. Use it to affirm something positive about yourself.

If you're a person who is easy-going and generally finds it difficult to speak up for yourself, you will find this exercise particularly beneficial. It helps you to connect your body with your mental energy so that your physical self and your emotional self are in alignment with your purpose and your will is, therefore, magnified. The exercise will take from five to twenty minutes.

Find a private space, preferably with a wood or carpeted floor. Think of a statement you need to affirm or own as the truth. It might be, "Yes, I can do that now!" or "No! Don't tell me what to do," Or Yes! I am free!" Imagine that you are a giant as you say or shout the words. Physicalize your statement by stomping on the floor for emphasis. Don't hurt yourself. Move slowly and thump like a giant. As you shout, use your arms to get your entire body into it. Move around the room. Keep shouting and stomping on the floor with each word. Fling your arms into the air. This is a sort of magnified tai chi exercise that moves you from thought to action by integrating your physical and emotional self with your mental self. It is better and more opening to your vulnerability to say as much as possible in the positive affirmation perspective as compared with saying "no."

The Self-Loving Exercise

This exercise is designed to communicate your love for yourself to your mind through its hard-wired connections with your body. It will fill you with the love that you may have been lacking in your life. Simply acknowledging a part of your body that needs love may bring up memories of an emotional injury that occurred long ago. If you feel resistance, you can do a contemplation or the Age Count-Back Exercise to discover the original cause of the block. You may need to repeat the exercise many times because you are dealing with your entire lifetime. It should take from five to forty-five minutes.

Lie down or sit comfortably in a chair. Your eyes can be open or closed. Slowly touch every part of your body and as you do, tell yourself that you love you. *Feel* happiness and joy. Speak the words aloud or just say them to yourself. As you touch each part, name it: "I love you, feet." "I love my legs," and so on. By doing this you are affirming your affection for all of yourself, bringing balance to your entire being, and resolving conflicts within your body. Often, old negative imprinted emotions will be stuck in or associated with particular parts of your body. Touching those parts will often reveal the block or negativity associated with something in your past. You need to release and change these negative associations and replace them with self-acceptance and understanding of your own unique beauty in order to be free from illness and live the best life you can. Any part of your body that resists allowing itself to be loved deserves contemplation. Many illnesses result from a lack of self-love, which can sometimes be physically isolated and located.

A variation on this exercise would be to give yourself an oil or lotion massage, feeling love for yourself and all parts of your body as you do the massage. This promotes sensuality, a quality from which many of us have grown detached.

The Emotional Block Searching Exercise

Parts of your body are literally affected by moments of strong, unresolved emotion that are later manifested as physical problems. Finding and releasing these physical manifestations of negative emotional energy will help you to achieve better health. The exercise should take ten to twenty minutes.

120

There are two ways to do this, and you can either combine or alternate the techniques. One technique is to sit in front of a mirror as you do a self-inventory. Because these blockages can lodge anywhere in your body, you might want to do this undressed. As you look at each part of your body—your eyebrows, elbows, fingers, etc., see how you feel about each one. Ideally, you should feel good about every part of your body. If you have a negative reaction to any part of you, you need to ask yourself why. Whatever your appearance or physical condition might be, you need to love all of you.

Another technique would be to lie down, close your eyes, and think your favorite color. Imagine it moving and spreading throughout your body starting with your feet. If the color is reluctant to move through any part of you, or if it changes color when it reaches a certain spot, you need to ask yourself why.

For example, you might discover that you don't like your knees. As you become aware of this, you might spontaneously recall that when you were in eighth grade someone made a disparaging remark about your knees. That remark is subconsciously affecting you to this day, making it difficult for you to express your emotions and make changes in your life. Affirm to yourself that implanting this self-criticism was a mistake, and use self-talk to tell yourself that you have beautiful and capable knees. Affirm that you can enjoy yourself and do anything you need to do with your knees. The key is always to use self-talk to correct any mistaken thinking from your past.

The Altering of Pain Exercise

This exercise will transmute any painful feeling—such as backache, headache, or the residual pain of an old injury—so that you will no longer perceive it as negative. It will take approximately fifteen to thirty minutes.

To do this you should be sitting comfortably or lying down. If the feeling isn't currently present, concentrate on the memory of the pain. If it is present, feel it for the moment just as it is. Don't react to it; just take your time and really feel it. Now, mentally increase the intensity of the pain. Notice how easy it is to do that. Then after a few minutes, let the pain, real or imagined, subside. Realize fully how you can use your mind to manipulate the pain sensation. You will probably notice that the pain is no longer as intense as it was when you began the exercise.

Now feel the pain merely as a sensation. Let it register at the point where it shows up in your body but stop calling it pain. It is just a sensation. Notice that as you re-label it a sensation, the perceived quality of pain is now diminished or gone. It becomes just a locus of attention. Now feel the energy of the sensation and let it be drawn out of your body and into space. Relax as you let the sensation disappear and leave you. Send love and joy into the area vacated by the pain. Now get up and take stock, making it a point to remember how well you converted your discomfort into another sensation and how you moved it out and away from your body.

We label many of our feelings good or bad, pain or pleasure, but when you reregister them as sensations you can often transmute them and move them around or out of your body.

The Color Absorption Exercise

Different wavelengths of light actually have different properties, and bringing different colors into your body will help to balance your inner state. You may, for example, find that you want to eat different fruits and vegetables on different days, depending upon their color. There are overlapping applications of energy that exist among the nutrition, color, and energy needs of your body and spirit. You'll find that you need to bring in different colors for different lengths of time on different days. You can do it throughout your day to create balance within yourself. The exercise takes between eight and fifteen minutes to complete.

Find a comfortable position and close your eyes. One by one, imagine each color of the rainbow (red, orange, yellow, green, blue, purple, then violet)—as well as black and white if you wish. First, consider the color, then take it into your mind so that you "see" it internally. Feel yourself pulling the color into your body, to the core of your being, in every cell, more and more with every breath. As you do this, you will know when you've soaked enough into yourself.

The Light-Breathing Exercise

This is a way to heal yourself. Although it isn't necessary, you may want to augment its benefits by actually sitting in a stream of light as you do the visualizations. Feeling the warmth of the light on your skin will increase the power of the experience. The exercise takes from fifteen to thirty minutes.

Sit comfortably and imagine a balanced, white stream of light entering your lungs with each breath you take through your nose. Hold your breath for a second, then exhale through semi-pursed lips. As you exhale, see the light leaving your lungs.

Now think of some part of your body that might need care—a spot that holds an old physical or emotional injury. With each breath you take, see the light going to that healing location. Focus on the white light pushing out the emotion or injury. When you feel done, breath the light into your entire body; imagine your body filling up with the white, healing and balancing light.

The Listening and Seeing Exercise

This is a method of becoming more aware of things outside yourself and heightening your overall awareness of the subtle energies in the world around you. You can do it in any position of circumstance from sitting on a porch swing to riding on a subway, but I suggest that you begin by doing it at home, either sitting or lying down. The exercise takes ten to twenty minutes.

Close your eyes and notice the sounds around you. Sense them at first with your ears, then see what you are hearing with your mind's eye. You might, for example, notice a clock ticking or a bird calling outside. Remain attentive to the physical space around you, investigating and concluding what is making each sound you bring into focus. Maybe you hear a buzzing. Is it a plane or a car? Listen again. Maybe the phone will ring; acknowledge it and let it go. Do you know who is calling? You'll find that the more you do this exercise, the calmer and more aware of your surroundings you'll become. It will increase your internal stillness as well as your awareness of your body, thoughts, feelings and world around you. It will allow you to listen to others with greater attention.

The Tactile Sensation Exercise

This exercise accesses the non-intellectual part of your brain in order to integrate your feeling and sensations with your thoughts. It also develops awareness and helps you to become more sensitive to the world around you. It takes from ten to thirty minutes.

Prepare a blindfold that securely covers your eyes and remove all breakable objects from the room in which you'll be doing the exercise. Pick a time when you won't be distracted. You can do the exercise without a blindfold if there's a room where you can be in total darkness; otherwise, the blindfold will ensure that you can't see your surroundings.

Walk around the room and feel whatever it is you bump into or touch, without exception. Walk and touch slowly, as if to let go of time.

"See" what you're feeling or touching with your skin. Notice textures and temperatures. Feel with your forearms or your face as you bump into things. Reach into the air and feel the space above you; touch the ceiling if it's within reach. Feel the movement of the air, your breath on your hand as you exhale. Feel the floor with your feet. Metals, plastics, and wood; chairs, tables, and lamps all have functions that you take for granted when you see them. Without your sight to tell how to label the item or what it's function is, you'll be experiencing them differently, opening yourself up to new experiences and awareness.

The Expression of Love Exercise

This is an exercise in sensuality that allows you to communicate intimately with the world around you. Sensuality relaxes the borders and defensive walls we normally put up around ourselves in the course of everyday life. It is a way for us to let go of the emotional control we exert on how others can touch us and how we express ourselves in return.

Sensuality can occur between you and another person or between you and a rock or a tree. It's a natural way to give and receive the love we all seek in our lives. The exercise is a safe and joyful way to develop your awareness of all that is "non-you," to help you express your vulnerability and open yourself up to receiving love. Take as long as you want with it and repeat it often.

You need to find a private room or outdoor space to do the exercise. Go around to every object in the space you've chosen and verbally express your love while touching the object. If you like, you can express your love in your thoughts without speaking it out loud, but be sure that you feel it throughout your body. Be sincere. As with all of life, it's what's in your heart that matters. When you do the exercise with living plants and trees, don't be surprised if you feel that you've heard them reply.

In Chapter Eight you'll find additional exercises to do while fasting in order to enhance the experience. The exercises in this chapter will also be enhanced if done while fasting. But, if you're not yet ready to fast, doing any of the exercises in this book will still help you to create more balance, openness, and health in every aspect of your life.

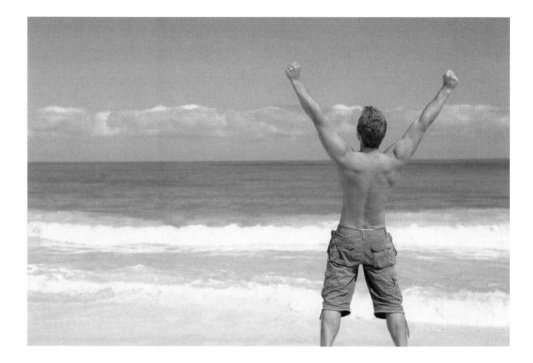

I Release,

I forgive,

I am Happy!

Chapter Seven

Release Anger and Depression; Embrace Self-Esteem, Responsibility, and Forgiveness

Both anger and depression are manifestations of blocked emotions or energy that need to be released and rebalanced so that you are able to live more freely, openly, and joyfully. We are taught by society that some emotions are "good" while others are "bad," but that isn't true. No emotion is necessarily good or bad in and of itself; what's bad is to suppress your emotions so that they build up inside you and create mental and physical pain. Instead, feel it and then let it go.

The opposite of holding onto anger and depression is to embrace self-esteem, take responsibility, and forgive both yourself and others for inevitable mistakes. To do that is a key to happiness and success. It is fundamentally important to realize that your beliefs create and put into action your emotional energy, which manifests in the physical world. When you have predominantly negative circumstances or emotions, you can look within to find the thought or belief that has generated and attracted those conditions.

What is Anger?

Anger is something we feel when we don't want to deal with a particular situation. It's a way for us to close-down. Often, we become angry when we think someone else is the source of our problems or because we don't want to accept another person's right to make decisions that are unacceptable to us. We think other people "make" us angry, but in truth, anger, like all emotions, is self-generated.

The more you are able to accept and respect other people's autonomy, the less you will tend to be angry with them. Instead of trying to force someone to do what you want or accept your point of view, allow yourself to be open and vulnerable enough to ask for what you want or need. You might not always get it, but you must understand that trying to run other people's lives instead of simply managing your own will almost always leave you frustrated and angry. In addition, your anger is likely to evoke an angry response, which means that you'll simply be bringing more anger into your life.

When you're angry, it means that you're closing down and have given up on finding other alternatives, but there are other alternatives, so long as you have the openness and patience to look for them and the faith that you will find them.

There are exercises in Chapter Six that can help you release pent-up anger and recapture the emotional openness you had as a child.

Are Your Choices Making You Depressed?

Depression is the result of subconscious choices and ways of reacting to situations in your past. Once you uncover them, you will be able to undo and change those choices. Everyone who is depressed has an original, self-generated, deeply embedded belief or thought that is coloring and directing his or her energy. All those who are depressed are gaining something from the depression; it may be protection from a particular vulnerability or a way of attracting attention without risk. Therefore, the "cure" resides within the person who is depressed, not in any outside person or circumstance. It requires looking within and focusing on the belief that is creating and driving the condition, which is what the person who is depressed wants to do least because it makes him or her feel even worse. (Electroconvulsive therapy, which uses electricity to temporarily reset the mind, statistically still has one of the best "cure" rates for depression.) Prescription medications and OTC herbal medications like St. John's wort might make people feel better chemically, but the people who take them then become less likely to want to uncover the original cause of their depression. I never prescribe anti-depressants, and I help patients who are already taking them to taper off gradually until they are drug-free.

Depression generally manifests as sadness, a low energy level, and lack of motivation. If you could put it in a test tube, label it, and analyze it, what would you add to fix it? Would you add loving and being loved? - humor, appreciation, forgiveness, a sense of self-worth? You can choose to fill yourself up with those qualities, but first you need to figure out how your previous choices got you depressed in the first place. It may take having to sit with the depression for a while, but eventually you will find the motivation to get yourself moving.

Maybe you saw so much anger growing up that you believe it's wrong to express anger. If so, you might need to rebel and release all that stored anger. Maybe you're afraid to express yourself because you lack a sense of self-worth. You don't have to be a genius to know that you're unhappy, unmotivated, and stuck, but you need to combine your emotional intelligence with your intellectual intelligence to gain self-understanding so that you can make new choices for yourself.

Sometimes we choose depression as a way to avoid accepting blame. If we believe others are hurting us, we may choose to hold onto the hurt instead of opening ourselves up to forgiveness so that we are once more free to accept love. We may think by doing that, the person who harmed us will recognize his wrong and begin to act differently. But that, unfortunately, could consign us to a lifetime of sadness as we wait for someone else to change. Or, conversely, if we see the suffering of others we may feel that we have no right to happiness ourselves. We need to be able to experience the pain and suffering of other people and still allow ourselves to feel and live our life, to affirm our own right to joy and peace. Whatever the complexity or appearance of depression it will trace back to one single self-generated belief. To change that belief, you have to be willing.

Use the contemplation techniques in Chapter Five to get to the source of your depression. Use the emotional exercises in Chapter Six to release negative energy and invite lightness into your life.

Self-Esteem, Responsibility, and Forgiveness Go Hand in Hand

Because your thoughts have power, what you think of yourself has the power to create who you are. If you strongly internalized negative thoughts and feelings about yourself in your past, you need to use your contemplation techniques to root out, release, and replace those thoughts and feelings with other, positive feelings of self-worth. Any thought that is not positive and self-affirming is self-destructive. That doesn't mean that you can't examine yourself objectively and realistically, but it does mean that you can't do it judgmentally.

To help heal yourself and increase your sense of self-worth, you can take responsibility for the way you live your life now and do things that are worthy. If you've made mistakes or been involved in negative situations in the past, free your conscious by forgiving yourself at the same time that you forgive everyone else for what they might have done to you.

Making the decision to do all that, can happen in an instant. Affirming your own value and rebalancing you feelings will take somewhat longer. At best you should be taking responsibility for everything you think, feel, say, or do, for your health, your successes, and your failures. Your health and happiness are yours to create every day.

Fasting releases the physician within.

Fasting breaks the cycle of unconscious eating and living.

Fasting naturally detoxifies the body and enhances the mind.

Chapter Eight

How to Fast

Once you have implemented all of the previous nine steps, you will be ready to get the most out of your fast. That said, you shouldn't embark on a fast without first consulting your physician, and you should never use fasting simply as a means to lose weight. Fasting breaks the cycle of eating for pleasure or eating for tension-release. The only permanent results you will get from fasting are what you discover through the self-exploration of your mind, emotions and embedded beliefs and are willing to change.

I also do not recommend fasting for growing children or adults and those fighting active infections.

There are many types of fasts: no water, water but no food, juice fasting, and specialty food fasting. I do not usually recommend any of these types of fasts. I recommend that you always have plenty of mineralized pure water to drink. I also recommend that you take supplements containing vitamins, minerals, and amino acids to provide for basic cellular function without the effects produced by the bulk of a regular meal. The body requires some amino acids each day to manufacture important neurotransmitters and enzymes.

Preparing for the Fast

By now you should have used the nutritional information in this book to shift your eating pattern toward natural, sugar-free, caffeine-free foods. You don't want to have to deal with the effects of coffee, sugar, or caffeine addictions or other types of imbalances during your fast.

Before you begin, there are a few items you'll need to purchase or make sure you have on hand.

1 Urine Chemstrips "SG" to test the specific gravity of your urine as well as to determine when the glycogen stores in your liver have been exhausted. These are sold at pharmacies and will allow you to check the concentration of your urine to determine whether or not you are properly hydrated. If your urine is too concentrated (the instructions will tell you how to determine this) you need to drink more electrolyte containing fluids.

2 A journal in which to record your thoughts and your dreams during your fast. Your dreams at this time can be very revealing if you know how to interpret them. Mary Summer Rain's book *20,000 Dreams* can help you to figure this out, or else you can simply record your thoughts, emotions and experiences. Looking at them later can reveal a lot about what your subconscious is telling you or experiencing.

3 Supplements including a high quality protein, vitamin, and mineral supplement.

4 Six-ounce cans of V-8 juice to be used sparingly for electrolyte replacement or you can use club soda with magnesium added to the volume.

5 A source of high quality pure water.

Beginning Your Fast

Remember a fast must be done with a positive mental attitude and positive emotions. Although you may be dealing with negative issues for a reason, the overall philosophy of the fast and your mood must be positive. You are trying to investigate and change yourself. The fast will give you greater clarity to do that.

Start by doing a one-day fast.

One-day fasts will introduce you to both the monitoring and the effects of a fast.

Keep yourself well hydrated and take a high quality vitamin but no other supplements. Keep your mind on positive things and try not to think about food or your mind will rebound after the fast. If you catch yourself thinking about food, take control of your mind and do any of the contemplative exercises or emotional energy exercises in Chapter Six.

Contemplation is the mental technique most useful during beginning fasts. Give yourself one issue to contemplate for the day.

After doing 3 to 5 one-day fasts you can go on to three-day fasts.

Three-day Fasts

The best time to do this is on a long weekend when you can start on a Friday and devote time to yourself. Make sure you have no other obligations during this time and can be primarily alone. To do this, you may have to plan your fast well in advance.

Fasting is primarily a solitary journey of self-discovery, but you may invite a friend or a psychologist to join you so long as he or she is aware of the purpose and techniques you are using. A person who is a good sounding board may be helpful during this time of contemplation and evaluation of your beliefs and emotional habits.

While you are fasting:

1 Each time you urinate, check your urine for specific gravity, and drink 6 to 8 twelve-ounce glasses of water each day. The glycogen stores in your liver will be used up in 24 hours and the Urine Chemstrips will show that you are ketoning, an indication that your body is burning fat for energy.

2 Take the vitamin and mineral supplements mentioned above.

3 You need 30 to 60 grams of protein each day or your body will begin to consume its own muscle tissue. To ensure that you are getting enough protein, prepare the following mixture.

Protein Supplement Mixture

Place about 8 pitted prunes, dried apricots, and dried figs in an 8-ounce glass (enough to fill the glass to the top).

Fill the glass with water and allow the fruit to soak in the refrigerator for 12 to 24 hours.

Transfer the rehydrated fruit and its liquid to a blender and add 1/2 teaspoon of Spirulina and 6 tablespoons of a high-quality protein supplement, one cut up banana and 1 cut up apple. Blend until smooth. Keep the mixture in the refrigerator and sip it intermittently throughout your fast to supply essential vitamins and amino acids.

Fasting for three days gives you the time to contemplate deeply, specific issues you want to become more aware of in your life. You can use any of the contemplative suggestions and emotional exercises in Chapters Five and Six to help you do this.

What is most important is to stay positive about whatever you are contemplating. You will discover much about yourself: your drives, thoughts, and emotional patterns. Your greater mind will answer your specific questions when you contemplate thoroughly.

Longer Fasts

After you've completed 3 to 6 three-day fasts you can begin to fast for 1 week and then eventually 2 weeks. I do not advise fasting for longer than 2 weeks, but fasting is such a personal experience you will have to judge for yourself how long you can or should fast.

As in all things, you can overdo it. Be sure to give yourself healthy food breaks between fasting episodes to fortify your body with the essential fatty acids and nutrients it requires for health. I recommend you take at least as much time off between fasts as the number of days you are fasting.

The more often you fast, the better your body becomes at it. That's why you repeat many shorter fasts before going on to longer ones. Your ability to monitor your fast for dehydration will improve as you become more familiar with your body's functioning.

For longer fasts, you need to replenish your electrolytes, and a V-8 juice can do that. I have a 6-ounce can every other day when I am fasting for longer than 3 days.

People commonly hit a three-day emotional wall that makes day three feel challenging. Maintain your positive consciousness and press forward with your mental contemplations and emotional exercises. You may be experiencing your thought processes and emotional tendencies objectively for the first time.

If you are fasting to lose weight, it is essential that you contemplate the thoughts, emotions, and lifestyle choices that have led you to overeat, not exercise, and so on. You need to determine how you handle stress and pleasure and discover the origins of your lifestyle choices. This is the true purpose of fasting: to find, alter, and balance your deepest beliefs, thought processes, and emotional responses. By doing that you will purify and bolster your will, faith, conviction, and consciousness.

Things You Can do to Enhance Your Fast

Full Body Massage

Any full-body massage can do wonders to help you release the tension from your body. During a fast in particular, you may experience great emotional release just from having part of your body massaged. This is because your elevated consciousness causes a heightened tendency toward energy-release.

Stretching

This exercise takes 15 to 30 minutes and is particularly good to do in the morning.

Be patient when you stretch; move gently and try not to stretch to the point of pain. If you do feel a painful spot during a stretch, breathe deeply into the area and relax as you exhale. Think about what you need to release from that particular area of your body. You may be surprised what specific thoughts come to you. As you exhale, affirm that you are thankful for any experiences in your past that have allowed you to be more loving, more sensitive, more open, and visualize the pain leaving your body along with the experience. You live in the now of loving.

Ending your fast

It is important to come out of a fast as if you had not been doing anything special. Your way of being should continue from fasting time to normal living time. Continue to be aware of your thoughts, and do not allow your mind to focus on food. You can control your thoughts by creating another subject for your mind to consider or by involving yourself in an activity or awareness that is not food-related.

You should come out of a fast if you cannot refrain yourself from thinking about food or if you cannot maintain a positive attitude during the fast.

The day after your fast you should consume mainly liquids and soft foods. When you begin to add other foods back into your diet they should be light and preferably vegetarian. If you are ready to dive into a steak you've probably got a lot more to contemplate.

When you reenter everyday life you will probably notice, where you didn't before, challenges to the discoveries you made during the fast. Almost everyone around you will have a tendency to want to keep you the way you were before in terms of your eating, lifestyle, and personality. This can be more or less of a challenge, depending upon your home and work relationships. Self-talk and affirmations will help you to continue on your forward journey. You may need to make major changes in your work or in how you choose to live your life.

Appendix A

Allergenic and Hypoallergenic Foods

Frequently allergenic foods considered best to eliminate when you are not sure of your body's compatibilities are: gluten (wheat and most grains), soy, cow milk, shellfish (crustacea), peanuts, strawberries, yeast, talc, lactose, artificial preservatives, artificial colors labeled like F, D and C # 5 or Yellow # 4, citrus, tree nuts, soybeans, chocolate, cocoa, beef, nightshade family (tomatoes, potatoes, eggplant, peppers, tobacco), sulfites, monosodium glutamate (MSG), sesame, alpha amylase and some fish.

In addition there are numerous common environmental allergies such as formaldehyde in new cabinets, furniture and other wood products, phthalates in plastics like Saran wrap, petroleum products, dust, latex and common seasonal plant allergens that can simulate food allergies. Names and derivatives of some food products:

Gluten is found in most all grains including: wheat, barley, rye, oats, kamut, spelt, triticale, couscous, bran, edible starch, semolina, farina, graham flour, malt, flour, durum, tabouli, macaroni, breads, pasta, cereals, hydrolyzed plant protein, paprika, baking powder, icing sugar, black pepper and modified food starch.

Cow's milk is also labeled: alpha casein, beta lactoglobulin, lactalbumin, bovine serum albumin, casein, caseinate, lactose, whey, curds and milk powder.

Eggs are also labeled ovomucoid, ovalbumin, lecithin, albumin and

143

ovovitellin.

Corn sources include fructose, zein, corn protein dextrose, glucose, corn gluten, corn starch, dextrin, dexin, dextrimaltose, corn alcohol (beer, bourbon, blended whiskeys, fortified wines, many liquors) and most caramel color.

Pineapple is also known as bromelain.

Barley is also called all-purpose flour, barley flakes, barley flour, enriched flour, malt and malted barley.

Beef derivatives are also known as bovine products, gelatin and gelatin desserts.

Papaya is called papain and meat tenderizer.

Coconut is also called MCT oil (medium chain triglycerides).

Peanuts are also in or are called goober peas, mandelonas, chili, vegetable burger, gravy, arachis oil and almond icing.

Tree nuts are found in pesto sauce.

Soy products are tofu, miso, natto, tempeh, soy infant formula, textured vegetable protein, soy milk, soy flour, soybean, and lecithin.

Diseases and conditions that can be associated with leaky gut, high protein diets or food allergies like gluten, but oft overlooked are: ADHD, autism, ADD, Development disorder, depression, epilepsy, migraine headaches, multiple organ failure, multiple sclerosis, alcoholism, ataxia, chronic brain syndromes, schizophrenia, intellectual impairment, difficulty concentration, dementia, eczema, unexplained rashes, bowel symptoms, brain fog, diarrhea, constipation, gas, irritability, anxiety, mood swings,

144

insomnia, ulcerative colitis, Crohn's disease, celiac disease, arthritis, asthma, autoimmune diseases, psoriasis, cankor cores, chronic sinusitis, itching, hives, nausea, sneezing, conjunctivitis and palpitations.

Hypoallergenic foods are considered best to eat in an elimination diet. They are: lamb, chicken, rice, sweet potato, carrots, rhubarb, asparagus, pears, banana, apricots, apple, sunflower oil and olive oil.

Appendix B

Foods that are Right for Your Blood Type

Blood type foods, while not individually always accurate, are a good place to start when determining the foods that are *most likely* compatible for your body. After doing an elimination diet, you may want to add the foods into your regimen one at a time from your blood type food group. Your individual reaction to the food is the final determinate whether you can eat that particular food without a problem, or not.

	Foods you can Have	Foods you Avoid
Blood Type A	Vegetarianism	Most meats and dairy, beans, wheat, ketchup, processed meat, corn oil, tomatoes, oranges, tropical fruit and most beverages.
Blood Type B	Red Meats, seafood, vegetables and pineapple.	Corn, lentils, peanuts, sesame seeds, buckwheat, wheat, poultry, beef, shellfish and rye.
Blood Type AB	Tomatoes, lamb, mutton, rabbit, turkey, cultured dairy products, eggs, vegetables and tofu.	Avoid same foods as A and B people. Cured or smoked meats, flounder, sole, pepper, corn products, oranges, and vinegar.
Blood Type O	Meat	Wheat, most grains, beans, legumes, breads, corn, brussel sprouts, cabbage, cauliflower, mushrooms, mustard greens, oranges, tangerines, alfalfa, night-shades, strawberries, coconuts, pickled foods, most beverages and dairy products.

Appendix C

Alkaline and Acidic Foods

In eating alkaline versus acid foods, it is generally considered better to eat towards the alkaline ph, or at least balance the more acidic foods that you eat with countering alkaline foods. For most people that means basically eliminating the most acidic foods from your diet unless they are combined with alkaline during that specific meal.

Vegetables

Most alkaline: lentil, onion, daikon, burdock, sweet potato, yam, kohlrabi, parsnip, garlic, asparagus, kale, parsley, endive, arugula, mustard greens, ginger root and broccoli

Moderate alkaline: potato, bell pepper, mushroom, cauliflower, cabbage, rutabaga, ginseng, eggplant, pumpkin, collard greens, brussel sprouts, beets, chive, cilantro, celery, scallion, okra, cucumber, turnip greens, squash, lettuce, jicama

Mild acid: spinach, fava bean, kidney bean, black-eyed peas, string bean, zucchini, chutney, rhubarb, split peas, pinto beans, white beans, navy beans, red beans, aduki beans, lima beans, mung beans, chard

Most acid: Soybean, carob, green pea, peanuts, snow peas, carrot, chick peas, garbanzo

Fruits

Most alkaline: lime, nectarine, persimmon, raspberry, watermelon, tangerine, pineapple, cantaloupe, honeydew, olive, mango

Mild alkaline: lemon, pear, avocado, apple, blackberry, cherry, peach, papaya, orange, apricot, banana, blueberry, raisin, currant, grape, strawberry

Mild acid: coconut, guava, dry fruit, fig, cherimoya, dates, plums, prunes, tomato

Most acid: cranberry pomegranate, jams, jelly

Grains

No very alkaline grains

Mild alkaline: oats, quinoa, wild rice, japonica rice

Mild acid: triticale, millet, kasha, amaranth, brown rice, buckwheat, wheat, spelt, kamut, teff, farina, semolina, white rice

Most acid: maize, barley, corn, rye, oat bran, processed flour

Nuts and Seeds

Most alkaline: pumpkin seed, poppy seed, cashew, chestnut, pepper

Mild alkaline: sesame seeds, almond, most seeds

Mild acid: pine nuts, tapioca, tofu,

Most acid: pistachio seeds, pecan, hazelnut, walnut, brazil nut

Oils

There are no very alkaline healthy oils

Mild alkaline: primrose oil, cod liver oil, avocado oil, coconut oil, olive oil, macadamia oil, flax oil

Mild acid: grape seed oil, sunflower oil, almond oil, sesame oil, safflower oil, pumpkin seed oil, canola oil

Most acid: chestnut oil, lard, palm kernel oil, cottonseed oil

Meat

There are no very alkaline meats

Mild alkaline: quail egg, duck egg

Mild acid: venison, fish, lamb, mutton, elk, shellfish, chicken eggs, wild duck, goose, turkey

Most acid: pork, veal, mussel, squid, beef, lobster, chicken, pheasant

Dairy

There is no very alkaline dairy

Mild alkaline: ghee (clarified butter)

Mild acid: butter, cream, yogurt, goat cheese, sheep cheese, cow milk, aged cheese, soy cheese, goat milk

Most acid: milk protein, cottage cheese, soy milk, processed cheese, ice cream

Spices and Herbs

Most alkaline: sea salt, baking soda, cinnamon, valerian, licorice, black cohosh, soy sauce

Mild alkaline: arnica, bergamot, echinacea, chrysanthemum, feverfew, goldenseal, lemon grass, willow bark, slippery elm

Mild acid: curry, vanilla, stevia

Most acid: nutmeg

Sweeteners

Most alkaline: molasses

Mild alkaline: rice syrup, succanat

Mild acid: honey, maple syrup

Most acid: saccharin, sugar, cocoa, aspartame

Beverages

<u>Most alkaline</u>: mineral water, kambucha

<u>Mild alkaline</u>: green tea, mu tea

<u>Mild acid</u>: kona coffee, alcohol, black tea

<u>Most acid</u>: coffee, beer, soda, malt

Vinegars

<u>There is no very alkaline vinegar</u>

<u>Mild alkaline</u>: apple cider vinegar, umeboshi vinegar

<u>Mild acid</u>: rice vinegar, balsamic vinegar

<u>Most acid</u>: white vinegar, acetic vinegar

Most antibiotics and psychotropic drugs are very acidic.

SOURCES Good for Reading:

The Inside-Out Diet by Mark E. Laursen MD, NMD, ABHM. More than the best diet book ever for permanent health & weight maintenance.

Healing from the Source by Dr. Yeshi Dhonden, the science and lore of Tibetan Medicine.

The Art of Listening by Bamberger & Brofsky.

Wonders of the Natural Mind by Tenzin Wangyal Rinpoche.

To Be Healed by the Earth by Warren Grossman, Ph.D.

Ayurveda - the Science of Self-Healing by Vasant Lad, BAMS, MA Sc.

Vibrational Medicine by Richard Gerber MD, an excellent reading on "Energy Medicine."

Aromatherapy by Daniel Penuel.

Spiritual Nutrition and the Rainbow Diet by Gabriel Cousens, MD.

You Can Heal Your Life by Louise L. Hay, a great standard reading on the connection of thought and emotion to physical ailments and disease.

Mary Summer Rain on Dreams by Mary Summer Rain and Alex Greystone.

Sunfood Cuisine by Frederic Patenaude is a very good recipe book and more on raw vegetarian cuisine.

Healthy Living by Linda Page ND, Ph. D.

Natural Health, Natural Medicine by Andrew Weil, MD.